LIVING
WITH A BRAIN
TUMOUR

"I have tried to live with
fear and not surrender to
its quiet, corrosive,
spirit-sapping power"

British Library Cataloguing in Publication Data
A record for this book is available from the British Library

ISBN 0 340 86428 1

Typeset in Minion by Avon DataSet Ltd,
Bidford-on-Avon, Warwickshire

Printed and bound in Great Britain by
Bookmarque Ltd, Croydon, Surrey

The paper and board used in this paperback are natural recyclable
products made from wood grown in sustainable forests.
The manufacturing processes conform to the environmental
regulations of the country of origin.

Hodder & Stoughton
A division of Hodder Headline Ltd
338 Euston Road
London NW1 3BH
www.madaboutbooks.com

Like a Hole in the Head

Living with a Brain Tumour

Ivan Noble

Hodder & Stoughton
LONDON SYDNEY AUCKLAND

To A, for all her wisdom and patience,
and our beloved children, M and F.

Contents

Editor's Note

Ivan Noble began writing this diary in September 2002. It was published on the BBC News website (bbc.co.uk/news) on a weekly, fortnightly or monthly basis, depending on the flow of events with his treatment. It is reprinted here largely as it was originally published. At the end of most of the chapters is a small sample of the thousands of e-mails sent in to the website by readers of the diary; all those included here have consented to having their e-mails reproduced. Also interspersed within the diary are four reflections subsequently written by some of those original readers who had particular perspectives on dealing with cancer. The BBC agreed with Ivan that all royalties it should make from this book would go to a charity of his choice: he selected Médecins Sans Frontières UK, registered charity number 1026588.

1
A New Beginning

My life and that of my family has just been turned upside down.

Last month I was a healthy young man in my mid-thirties, looking forward to working part-time, taking care of our baby daughter and making plans for next year. Now I have just been told that I have a fast-growing tumour inside my brain.

Reading between the lines I understand it is something an older man would have little chance of beating. With youth, determination and a lot of support on my side, I intend to be luckier.

The discovery began with a week of increasingly unpleasant headaches, bad enough to wake me early but fading off into the morning and then coming back in the evening to leave me sleepy.

By the end of the week they were strong enough to make me sick and I was with my GP, who sent me to Accident and Emergency at the local hospital, where the care was impressively fast.

Within hours I had a CT (computed tomography) scan of my

head and it was at that point that a charming young doctor told me they had found 'something interesting'. Stupidly, I felt flattered.

Brain tumours are very unusual at my age, he said, and it was much more likely that I had picked up a nasty infection on a recent reporting trip to West Africa. That infection had probably found its way to my head and was causing a swelling which needed dealing with swiftly. A minor brain operation, lots of antibiotics and rest would do the trick.

On a bank-holiday weekend, the staff had to work hard to find a neurosurgical hospital bed for me. But they did and, after a short ambulance ride and a few anxious hours, I was operated on at two in the morning by a cheerful and confidence-inspiring surgeon.

At nine I got the news I had not wanted. There was no bug, no infection, just a little fluid and what looked like a tumour. It was going to take four days to analyse the small fragment they had removed.

Four days later an uncomfortable doctor gave me the news. 'There are no good brain tumours to have,' he said, 'but if there were, yours would not be one of them.' But it was not the end of the road, he said.

He left us to interpret that and I was allowed home.

Less than a day after hearing my diagnosis in the grim 'room of doom' interview suite, I was with a consultant oncologist discussing my treatment. He told me exactly what I wanted to hear: 'You've got everything to fight for, and we're going to throw the book at your tumour.'

The shock has been enormous. I have spent many hours wandering around, starting to make cups of tea or fill the dishwasher, and then forgetting what I had started doing. And the fear, for some days, was paralysing. I often had the urge just to lie down and sleep. But, as the days have gone by, I have my nerve again. Talking to friends, family and anyone who would listen has helped. So too have all the medical friends and acquaintances who have provided encouraging titbits of information.

We have asked many questions of the doctors and that, too, has always helped. I have not asked what my chances are and I do not want to know, for the simple reason that I think no one knows. The doctors understand what I have and how to treat it, but no one can know how well the treatment will work. All the statistics in the world will not tell them what is going to happen to me, and I am grateful for the uncertainty and hope that provides.

The National Health Service has been very good to me. It saved my life when I was twelve years old and it was there for me this time when I needed it. Its staff were without exception professionally excellent and there were many instances of kindness and compassion for which I will always be grateful. But as an organisation it has now delivered one big disappointment. I need radiotherapy with some urgency, and the best estimate I could get from the NHS was a six-week wait. I have medical insurance through my employer and I am lucky enough now to have started privately arranged treatment on Wednesday, less than two weeks after my diagnosis. There are thousands of cases like mine every year in this country; most people will not have that option.

My blessings are countless and I could not be in a better position for what I have to face now. I am determined to beat the tumour and to see my little girl grow up.

Thursday 19 September 2002

The noise of the radiotherapy machine is the best thing.

I have been in four times now and each time I find it inspiring. It starts just after the technicians leave the room to go behind their screen and it lasts for about half a minute. It is a powerful combination of ticking and shushing and I am convinced it is doing me the power of good.

A friend said to try to imagine the tumour melting as I am being irradiated so I try to picture a science film I once saw about how the body gets rid of cells it has finished with. I see the radiation hitting my squiggly little tumour cells, shattering their DNA and forcing them to abandon their takeover bid in my head. I think it is working. I have another twenty-six sessions to go.

The whole thing is utterly painless and from entering the hospital to leaving it again takes around twenty-five minutes, except on the days when I have to talk to the doctor and the nurses. A plastic helmet moulded in the shape of my head makes sure that I am positioned correctly on a metal stretcher each time I go in. The technicians line up the powerful X-ray machine that delivers the radiation dose and then they fire off two half-minute blasts, one from the side of me and one from behind. Each is designed to target the quadrant of my head where the tumour is lurking.

My doctor says that he and I will not know how well the radiotherapy has worked for a month or two after it ends, perhaps in December. We will not be able to scan the tumour and see what size it is until then because it will probably swell and scar first. Because it is such a nasty specimen, I will move on to chemotherapy – a drug treatment to poison what is left of the tumour – before we know any results from the first round. My doctor is confident I am strong enough to cope with the side effects.

The wonderful thing is that I feel so fit now. I am being given steroids to counteract swelling around the tumour and, ever since I have been taking them, I have had no headaches or pain at all. They also boost my energy and appetite, though they do seem to make me slightly hyperactive too. As time goes on I can expect to start losing my hair and feeling more tired, but I am told that the treatment of brain cancers can be less of a burden than for cancers elsewhere in the body.

The tissue of a healthy adult brain is no longer growing. Both radiotherapy and chemotherapy fight cancer because they destroy cells which are growing, especially ones which are growing quickly. So, with luck, the tumour gets zapped and the healthy bits of my brain stay that way.

The more I learn about the treatment, the less frightened I feel. And fear really has given way for me to think about the number of things we have to organise. Treatment could affect my fertility, so I have decided to deposit sperm. I have never made a will, so I need to do that. And I want to make sure that I get on the national register for consent for organ donation and medical research. I might face more surgery down the line and it is not without risks. Then there are the little indulgences like buying a new printer for our computer.

I think it is much tougher for the people close to me than it is for me. I am loved, cared for and receiving excellent treatment. I have no choices to make, just the job of getting on with the task in hand and spending my time well.

I fell in love with the city in which I live when I moved here four years ago, and over the past two weeks my partner and I have had some time to enjoy it and do things we would not otherwise have had time for.

I am deeply grateful to everyone who has e-mailed me over the past week with encouragement and suggestions. The warmth and optimism have been overwhelming and I want to think with my colleagues about how best to make sure I am not the only beneficiary of all the advice.

I am grateful also to the Inland Revenue, Britain's tax collection authority, who wrote this week asking me to estimate my income for the tax year 2003 to 2004. That made my week. I must write back tomorrow.

Tuesday 1 October 2002

I have just had my tenth dose of radiotherapy and I have twenty more to go. I have to wear a transparent plastic shell on my head to keep it in the right place for the technicians to line up the beam. It is not uncomfortable and I only have to wear it for about five minutes. It has holes for my eyes and nose and clamps at the back to hold me still. I am hoping to hang on to it when I have finished.

This week I have dipped my toe in the waters of medical information on the Internet and have given myself a real fright. It made me think really hard about how much I want to know about my tumour. I was browsing at four in the morning, wide-awake as I sometimes am from the steroids I have to take. I came across a site where a patient who said he had the same tumour as I have described was asking a doctor how many people with our condition are alive three years after diagnosis.

'None' was the reply he quoted.

I do not know whether there is any truth in what he says but, of course, it terrified me. Until now I have been working on the assumption that however bad my chances might be statistically, they are not zero and therefore I have everything to fight for. Not just a relatively long and pain-free illness, but perhaps a real long-term remission. I decided not to believe what I had read.

It was an anecdote among many, and for every time I have heard something like that, I have heard ten stories of people surviving years and even decades. I am sceptical that anyone really is 'given months to live', anyway. It seems such an impossible thing to predict that I cannot imagine any doctor committing themselves, unless a patient really insisted.

I have decided to steer clear of medical websites for the time being. I am fit and well and strangely very happy at the moment, so I am just going to ignore them. It is wonderful that so much information is available and that patients can be as well-informed

6

as they want to be. But it is very difficult to filter that information. It is not possible to start to search the Net and hope to see only encouraging news. Along with the details of therapies, diets and clinical trials, there is cold, clinical information out there about how many people die and how they die. Link leads to link and it is easy to terrify yourself.

The great luxury I have is that my partner is a biologist who works in cancer research. It has been a massive shock to her suddenly to have her career made intensely personal in this awful way, but in the circumstances, her knowledge and contacts are very useful for me. She has the unenviable task of sifting through information on treatments and giving me the positive stuff, for which I am very grateful.

We think that the bottom line is that there is much we and my doctors do not yet know about my tumour. In time we will know how tough it is going to be to kill, but only in time. There is plenty for us to be busy with before then.

One more thing I read on the Net was that my feelings of almost enjoying the therapy are not uncommon. Many other patients also get a real boost out of starting treatment and it is not uncommon to feel a bit of an emotional low at the end of the radiotherapy, simply because it is a shock to be doing nothing and waiting to see what has happened after being the subject of such intensive care and attention for weeks. I know that come late next month I am going to miss my daily trips, even if by then I am tired and patchy on top as a result of them.

I have suffered only one major side effect from the whole cancer experience so far, and that has been financial. Anyone who knows me will know my obsession with gadgetry, particularly any kind of gadgetry which can be connected to other gadgetry and made to do something pointless but hard to configure. Connecting satellite navigation receivers to old laptops running obscure operating systems and simultaneously linking to a PDA (Personal Digital Assistant) is my idea of recreational heaven.

But there is a natural barrier to pointless gadget acquisition formed by the fact that there is always something new coming along and it is usually better to wait three months and get the next model, or this model when it is no longer at its bleeding-edge price, or the second generation one with the drivers that actually work.

Being diagnosed with a brain tumour blows that restraint out of the water. Online retailers of the world, rejoice!

From: Simon Lawrence, UK

I had testicular cancer three years ago – though it's all clear now. But I can relate to your comments about the radiotherapy, I had fifteen sessions, each with two thirty-second doses. I found it funny watching the nurses scamper out of the room to hide and then hear that click followed by a low hum. I wish you all the best, take care.

From: David, England

I am thirty now and was diagnosed with malignant tumours about six years ago. Over the course of a year I had a series of operations and then was put on a year of chemo. At the time I was given a fifty-fifty chance of making it through. I am now as healthy as a bean, although I still go for annual check-ups. Keep a positive attitude, I have done a lot of Web-based research about cancer and it seems that those with a positive attitude

against fighting this irritating disease
show a much better chance of beating it
than those who are dejected and depressed.

From: M Brimacombe, Devon, UK

Well done for having the courage to tell
people about this and not skulking in the
shadows. It gives everyone hope.

From: Marc, South Africa

I was diagnosed with a benign tumour
bigger than a snooker ball in my neck and
I have just had it removed a few days
ago. I still carry the stitches and won't
be able to speak properly for the next
few months. But for me, life is not about
the destination; it's about appreciation
and sheer joy of the little things.
Celebrate the beauty of humanity with
those close to you and remember that life
is beautiful.

From: Doug, UK

About a month after I got engaged, aged
thirty-two, I was diagnosed with a tumour
in almost the same location as yours.
Luckily mine was benign and non-invasive
(I suppose it was 'one of the good
ones'). About four months after I got
married, I had the tumour removed and
thankfully have made a full recovery. All
I can say is, stay positive and work on

your own wellbeing. If you are not
selfish, then you need to be – your
energies should be concentrated on
staying physically and emotionally at the
top of your game. No doubt you have heard
of Lance Armstrong's book *It's Not About
the Bike* – he was given a 30 per cent
chance, and look what he's done since
then.

2

Understanding My Tumour

A great clump of my hair fell out almost all at once on Saturday. We went out into the garden and shaved off the rest to keep things even. I was happy. It felt like something was happening. The radiation must be giving the tumour a hell of a time.

Instead of reading scary Web pages, I have been reading about how cancer starts. Some types of cancer run in families, but I was glad – for my daughter's sake – to learn that tumours like mine do not.

They are more common in men than women, and more common in people older than me, but that is about all we know. Lots of people have asked if I think I got the tumour because I use a mobile phone a lot. I have to say that right at the moment I think not. The current evidence is inconclusive and I think my tumour is in the wrong place in any case.

The fact is that no one really knows yet what causes cancers like mine. Yet cancer researchers do understand a great deal about how the disease arises in the body and they are learning more by the day. Two years ago I read a book called *One Renegade Cell* by Robert Weinberg, a cancer research pioneer. It opened my eyes to the wonderful process by which the human body keeps itself cancer-free for most of most people's lives.

Cancer is frightening but it becomes less so the more you understand what it is. The human body needs to replace cells from time to time. We are constantly growing new skin, for example, and all over the body, tissue needs replacing as we get older. When cells in the body need to multiply to grow new ones, they use instructions contained in their DNA. In a healthy body, they make enough new cells for the job in hand and then they stop. Cancer is simply what happens if this process gets out of control and the cells keep on growing without stopping.

My brain tumour is no alien invader which needs a name for it to be cursed and cast out. It is just a lump of cells which has gone wrong and forgotten how to stop growing. I am hoping the large doses of radiation it is currently receiving might jog its memory.

It is reassuring to know how many safety mechanisms the body has to prevent cancer. A cell's DNA can easily be damaged. When new cells are made, the DNA from the parent cell is sometimes copied wrongly – or chemicals like those in tobacco smoke can damage the DNA, as can radiation.

This happens all the time, but the body is very good at spotting it and killing off damaged cells before they have a chance to divide and pass on copies of their faulty information. Very occasionally in a person's life, a damaged cell survives and starts creating copies of its damaged self. Even then, there are safeguards that ensure that those cells do not develop into a tumour.

Four to seven different mechanisms are at work in some way inside the body, wiping out damage and keeping us healthy. Not unless they all fail does anyone get cancer. The failure of any one of these mechanisms is unlikely and happens randomly.

The statistical truth is that most of us succumb to something else long before all those safety locks fail. People in families where cancer is common simply have one or two safety locks off already. They have inherited one or two mutated or faulty safety-lock genes. But they are not for a second doomed to get cancer – they simply have a higher chance than other people.

Cancer strikes at random, but of course there is plenty you can do to reduce the chances of any of your safety locks coming off. Robert Weinberg makes no bones about the best way: stop smoking, or do not start. Tobacco smoke contains a potent cocktail of nasty chemicals, any one of which can easily be the trigger for one or more of those safety-lock genes failing.

Oh, and wear sunscreen.

3

Time Pressures

I heard from my doctor today something I had already decided to believe. He told me I do have a chance of beating the tumour. Another doctor, a friend, told me the same a few days ago. It is a relief. I have been too scared to ask whether my treatment is really an attempt to destroy the tumour or just to slow it down and prolong my life as long as possible. I do not care how big or small the chance of full remission is. It is my chance and I will seize it.

I learned more about how my radiotherapy was planned from one of the radiographers today. Calculating the angle at which to aim the X-ray beams at my head was a complex business. The radiographers have done a wonderful job. Two beams of X-rays are – slowly but surely – dosing the tumour with radiation to disrupt its growth. But they are carefully aimed to miss vital areas of my lower brain.

On the treatment planning form are two boxes for the doctor to describe the type of radiotherapy. One is marked 'radical'; the

14

other is marked 'palliative'. I was delighted to see that on my form 'radical' was ticked.

The radiation dose is very high. My healthy, non-cancerous brain cells should be able to stand it and return to normal in the end, but we hope the cells in the tumour will wither under the assault, just like my hair has done.

It is falling out all over my head now. The left and back, where the X-rays enter my head, fell out last week. Now the right and top, where the two beams leave my head, are also coming away. I have a fringe of stubble and not much else.

Given that everyone is taking such good care of me, I have had to think about what I can do to support the process. I have little trouble maintaining a positive attitude, universally recommended as the best medicine, but I have had to think hard about all the other remedies.

I have had dozens of pieces of advice from friends, family and people who have read this diary. Some have been unconventional, like the person who drank large spoonfuls of curry powder in a glass of water each day with the result that the tumour left the body of its own accord. I am a great curry fan but I can't foresee my tumour crawling down my neck or out of my nose.

A lot of the advice makes good sense to me. I have tried to put a sensible diet together, cutting right back on red meat, dairy products, sugary foods and my beloved pork pies. Instead I am eating stacks of antioxidant fruit and vegetables – apples, tomatoes, broccoli and beans. Fish has taken the place of steak and mince.

I am not sure whether eating better will make any difference but it has turned out to be less of a wrench than I expected.

Many people said various forms of visualisation would help me beat the cancer. My mother is a big believer in these things and she taught me to imagine the tumour melting under the radiation. I now see in my mind a full colour picture of it gasping its last each time I go under the machine. Other people have told me to try relaxation techniques and I can certainly see the sense in them.

Having a condition like this does generate a powerful urge to get things done, and I often work myself into a hectic frenzy, which cannot be good for me and is definitely not easy to live with. I have not found anything yet but I am thinking t'ai chi or yoga might help.

I hope the cells in my tumour are starting to die now. If they are, then my body has the job of getting rid of them. So I need to make life as easy as possible for my kidneys and liver. I am downing two litres of water a day, trying to walk more to keep up my metabolic rate and taking an extremely moderate approach to alcohol and coffee – normally two great pleasures in my life.

I am surprised to find myself feeling so open to all these things. Under normal circumstances I would be more sceptical. But I do have the urge to do everything I can to swing the odds in my favour and not simply be a passive recipient of treatment. I have to draw the line at apricot kernels, though. They are recommended by many sources as containing a vitamin which attacks cancer in the same way as vitamin C attacks scurvy. What put me off was a medical research paper describing the effects they had in a fairly substantial number of patients. None showed any measurable progress, but a substantial proportion suffered toxic side effects as their bodies released cyanide from one of the components of the kernels.

For the moment I am hoping a more conventional poison will help. In just over a week, I finish radiotherapy and after that, chemotherapy starts.

Monday 21 October 2002

I am running down the home straight of the first lap of my treatment. I have only four radiotherapy sessions left to go, though it will be many weeks before I learn what effect the treatment has had. The prospect of starting chemotherapy in less than three weeks is daunting.

The drugs I will take are very powerful and although I have had plenty of reassurance from my doctor about how well I will tolerate the side effects, I cannot help being slightly nervous. So far I have felt 100 per cent fit. But now I have stopped taking the steroids I was given to control swelling in and around my brain.

One of the many side effects of steroids is that they do tend to keep you awake. Deprived of the steroid boost, the side effects of my daily dose of radiation are starting to kick in. I often feel tired during the day and doze off for five minutes now and then, sometimes on my way to the hospital. It is not alarming to feel the tiredness coming on. Like having my hair fall out, it is a sign that something is happening. Now that my various bald patches have all combined, I look like a poor man's Ronaldo. I'm happy I've had such an easy ride so far and am looking forward to trying to get away for a few days in the gap between the radiotherapy ending and the chemotherapy beginning.

Now I am off all medication apart from the cocktail of vitamins I take every morning. And healthy eating is proving far less of a trauma than one might expect for a man whose first choice is steak and chips.

There has been plenty to think about. Suddenly I cannot ignore all the news stories about the latest advances in cancer research. It is awkward to hear of research results which are naturally good news but will not actually mean a direct improvement in survival rates for several years. Not everything billed as a 'breakthrough' feels that way when you plan ahead in weeks and months, not years.

There are many good reasons why the worlds of science and drug development move slowly, but they are less easy to accept when time is such a precious thing. Every week someone comes up with a way of improving the treatment of a particular type of cancer and every week the odds shift a little more in favour of the human race and against cancer in all its forms. But I cannot help wishing they would shift more quickly.

Our little girl turned nine months old this week. She has four new teeth to go with the two she already has, and she's learned to pull herself upright and stagger around holding on to whatever is in her grasp.

I'm delighted she's developing so quickly and I am proud of the way she takes on the world with such energy and enthusiasm. Thinking about her future, though, is the thing I find hardest.

Despite all my optimism, I have to bear in mind the possibility that the tumour might in the end get the better of me. I am determined that it will not, but I cannot escape thinking now and then that she might grow up without me. That is the one single thing that leaves me fighting back tears. But for every time that happens, there are ten more that she and her mother make me crack a smile.

Ten more times when I realise what exactly I am fighting for.

I am touched, encouraged and grateful for the response to my diary. Receiving encouragement and tales of recovery from all over the world is a privilege most cancer patients do not have. It is a great source of strength. I will do all I can to repay the generosity with a happy ending.

From: Steve, UK

Out of the blue I had a fit, aged twenty-four, which led to the discovery of a brain tumour. Radiotherapy did little to help and as I was beginning chemotherapy I was told I probably had three to eighteen months left to live. Over seven years later I'm still here, happier and fitter than before the original diagnosis.

I'm a teacher (alas not in the state sector) and financial pressures have made me work throughout. I think this was probably good therapy though I was treated disgracefully by management at the treatment stage. There is a strong need for more statutory protection here. The last thing I needed while coping with the trials of radiotherapy was to be told that my position would be 'ominous' if I took time off.

For me it's the fatigue that's been my greatest problem – and the one that seems most difficult for others to really understand. As 'we all get tired' it often doesn't register that this sort of on-going, life-changing fatigue is of a quite different order.

Short-term memory is a bit of a problem. I can still recount my school class register of twenty-five years ago, but frequently forget whether I've already told the same story to the person I'm talking to the day before, causing me to preface most of what I say with 'I might have already mentioned but . . .' which is a bit tiresome. Also, in speech, it's sometimes difficult to get the right word in time, leading either to awkward pauses mid-sentence or the mind making a frantic stab for the nearest alternative, usually grabbing something that sounds similar (a 'clang' mistake I'm told) rather than meaning the same. So long as

I'm aware this is happening, as it's
happening, I've learnt to find it an
irritation rather than a worry. And
because I type so slowly it's not a
problem with the written word!

Overall the biggest surprise is that I
would not have expected to be able to
cope as well as I have. Good friends have
been essential here. A common and well-
intentioned adjective showered upon me
over the years is 'brave'. I'm no braver
than the next man. In fact I have been
known to jump into the arms of whoever
I'm talking to at the sound of a car
back-firing so brave am I. It's really
not been a matter of courage, much more
it's been a clear-headed view that if
time is limited the worst thing I could
do would be to wallow and waste it.
Occasionally this means 'brave faces' but
usually it's just getting on and living a
life.

From: Hilary Dibble, UK

I'm in remission from breast cancer,
sixteen months after completing chemo and
radiotherapy. I can identify with all you
say – and though they tell us that
thinking positively may not help your
clinical symptoms, it certainly helped me
cope with the treatment. I worked short
days throughout my treatment, except for
when I was at my most vulnerable after

chemo - and at times I felt as though my
brain had been swapped for cotton wool.
But I've now been back at work full time
for more than six months - and I promise
you it does get easier. I will keep my
fingers crossed for your scan in March -
just make the most of all that life can
offer in the meantime. I am not at all
confident that my cancer has gone for
good and I now focus much more on
enjoying life to the full.

From: Karen James, UK

Your comments help me understand better
the radiotherapy my brother Richard is
about to start. His diagnosis mirrors
yours. Your fighting spirit is
encouraging, keep it up!

From: Alex Newbery, Scotland

At twenty-three, I was diagnosed with an
inoperable brain tumour spreading down
into the brain stem (the bit they can't
chop out) and was given a 3 per cent
chance of surviving an operation. After
two operations at Charing Cross in
London, I am now thirty-two and married
with three kids.

They've crippled it so that it should
grow slowly enough that when it needs
operating on again (who knows, maybe ten
years), they will know enough to clear it
with a 'dissolve in water' kind of pill.

4
Future-gazing

Last week I met a group of other people with brain tumours and heard some incredible stories. One woman had had a tumour for thirty years. Hers was not the same kind as mine, but her story was inspiring nevertheless.

Another woman told the story of her husband, who has had a tumour similar to mine for nine years and is in good health and great spirits. But at the same event I also stumbled across the very information I had been trying to avoid – the survival rate for my tumour.

I do not want to go into details, but let me just say that it was no great boost for me.

But it is interesting to look at what survival rates actually mean. Doctors often deal with median survival periods. They are simple statistics which indicate the length of time it takes for half of the patients with a certain condition to die. So if the median survival rate for cancer X is one year, one would expect fifty out of 100 patients to be dead by the time a year had passed since their symptoms began.

Many years ago, a far better writer than I wrote about this, as readers of this diary have pointed out. Stephen Jay Gould was diagnosed with a rare cancer and told that the median survival period was eight months. He wrote *The Median is Not the Message* and lived another twenty years. Closer to home, a nurse at the meeting I attended mentioned a patient with my condition who was diagnosed in 1985. That patient is still well.

There is plenty for me to aim for, but I have to say that the experience of spending a whole day thinking about my cancer and dealing with some hard and gruesome facts left me scared and tired.

Doctors face a very difficult task when they decide how much to tell patients. They have to think about keeping a patient's spirits up and preserving the will to live, but at the same time they may feel that depriving a patient of accurate information on their condition deprives them of the right to make well-informed decisions. I would not like to be in their shoes, nor would I have liked to be in the shoes of the registrar who had to give me my diagnosis.

I followed up a tough day of tumour facts with a visit to the neurosurgeons who did the emergency operation on me at the end of August. The occasion for the meeting was to see how my scar had healed, but I ended up hearing more than I had hoped about the difficulty of managing a tumour like mine.

I felt my optimism ebbing away and started thinking the thoughts I try to avoid – the ones about things like what to put in my final letters to my family. Now I am glad I have had to face up to the hard facts and figures.

My spirits, like those of most people, are swung by fatigue and the weather. As I write, it is a beautiful, clear autumn day and I am well rested, happy and positive.

It may be my imagination, but I feel that I am getting better and that my vision is improving together with my other symptoms. The neurosurgeons say that even if I do very well, I will never regain the sight I have lost on my right side. I am not so sure.

The next step for me is chemotherapy, beginning on 6 November. We will go from trying to kill my tumour with powerful X-rays to trying to poison it with powerful drugs.

In the meantime, we are scanning the websites of the discount travel agents.

Thursday 31 October 2002

Finishing radiotherapy has meant having the chance to travel. We have just come back from a weekend in Berlin, and, by the time this is published, we should be in Portugal for the first time, exploring the southern coast.

Getting away was wonderful and for much of the time I could completely forget the tumour. Berlin was my home for two years in the 1980s and I felt like my old self again, excited by a place where so many layers of history are still raw and exposed.

My little daughter saw plenty of new faces and took it all in her stride, laughing back at everyone who smiled at her and charming other passengers on the plane home. I hope that she will like Portugal as much as Germany.

We will be back home in time for my chemotherapy to start on 6 November.

The more my spirits lift, the more I can conceive of longer-term plans. Many of them are mundane, but they are plans I would have been scared to contemplate when I was still in hospital. I love life, and I want more of it. There are, too, plenty of people who say having faith in a future is the road to recovery.

Faith is a question which comes up again and again. People from all over the world have e-mailed to say that they are praying for me, as have friends and family.

I am touched that they are and I am grateful for their thoughts, even though I am not religious myself. I was brought up without religion and the only contact I had with it was at school, where it seemed to be largely a disciplinary tactic.

It was not so much that I rejected religion as that I never got to know it in the first place. Some very good friends are believers, but it seems to be so much a part of the culture they grew up in that it would feel odd for me to attempt to travel their road.

I would not describe myself as lacking in faith in any case. I have an enormous faith in the fundamental good in people. Humans are social animals who would long since have become extinct if they had not looked after each other. Their urge to understand and control the world, displayed to me daily by one particularly young example of the species, has led them to develop the science and medical technology that gives me cause for hope in the first place.

There is a new, experimental treatment for my condition which has shown promise in trials and is now entering what are called phase three trials, where people are selected randomly from a group and given either the new treatment or a placebo. The results of this trial will take years to come through, but the treatment could be licensed in time to help me if I do get a remission and then relapse.

The fatigue which follows radiotherapy is really starting to unfold now. I was never a person who found it easy to get up early, but now it is a battle. I need to sleep once or twice during the day and if I do not manage it, then I am very sleepy and very poor company in the evening. The tiredness is not debilitating, but I cannot ignore it indefinitely. Days have always seemed too short to me and it is frustrating to have to sleep when there is so much to be done.

So, time to deal with the first item on the list – finding a bucket and spade.

From: Marjorie Cliff, USA

Our prayers are being winged to you from
the High Desert of Southern California.
As a transplanted Londoner, and the
recipient of a donated heart in 1994, I
am acutely aware of what a life-
threatening disease can do to one's
entire life. I have lived the past eight
years with the miracle I was given, but
nevertheless I have learned to savour
each day as though it were the last. May
you be blessed as I have been, and enjoy
many more years.

From: Doug, UK

I work too hard – I miss my children – I
save for a pension – I have absolutely no
idea of the gifts that are with me. My
prayers are with you – my energy's with
you – my will's with you. Live long!

From: Karim Moukaddem, Spain

Don't stop writing even when you are
totally recovered. When everything turns
out well (*inshallah*) we would love to
share the happier times with you. The way
you opened up yourself to all of us has
shown us that deep within us there is a
tremendous force at our disposal, if only
we could see it.

From: Cathy, USA

As a nurse, I have seen a positive
outlook accomplish good things for
patients. If you are comfortable with
God, and have great faith, that is an
immeasurable asset, as well. Not only is
there the reassurance and comfort now,
but also there is no worry for your
future. Rest well, eat well, and may God
hold you in the palm of his hand.

From: Yukio Tsuchida, Holland

I practise life philosophy of Nichiren
Buddhism in Soka Gakkai. I want to say to
Ivan to chant *nam myoho renge kyo*.

From: Stanislas Hutten Czapski, UK

Time and again I forget how fortunate I
am to have a healthy family. And when I
do that, I make life overcomplicated. I
hope to help you with positive thoughts –
be sure you have already helped me. I too
have a young family and stopped smoking
three days after I read your diary.

5

Internal Struggle

Four white capsules, each with a smart blue double stripe, have now joined the vitamins and anti-epilepsy drugs on my daily menu. These powerful chemotherapy drugs are designed to mop up cancerous cells left behind by the radiotherapy. There are also two tiny white pills, one triangular, the other circular, to stop the chemotherapy making me feel sick.

So far there have been no side effects but then I took them only four hours before writing this. I am still tired as a result of the radiotherapy and I get the odd twinge of a headache, enough to keep me worrying but no more.

The plan is that I take the chemo tablets for five days then rest for twenty-three days before taking another set. There will be four sets in all. The drugs are fiendishly expensive and I am lucky to have them.

I saw the doctor and he said we would not do another scan to see how the tumour has responded to treatment until next year. I know that the run-up to that scan will be nerve-wracking and I am happy that it will not be for a while.

It felt reassuring to see the doctor and the rest of the staff at the hospital again. Their manner is so infectiously positive. And, despite the obvious attractions of a Mediterranean break, it felt good to be back home when we arrived on Tuesday. On this last trip away I had a bit too much time to think, and again ended up in the internal struggle to stay positive. That really has been the hardest thing so far.

When I try to visualise the long-term future, sometimes it works but sometimes I just end up seeing all the hurdles I will have to clear. A great remedy for beating encroaching gloom is to focus on someone else's cares and problems. But sometimes it is hard to put this theory into practice and easy to slip into self-absorption. When that happens, it is very easy to start seeing graphs, curves and depressing images.

I have been very lucky. Other people with brain tumours have to grapple with seizures, which I have so far been spared. Depending on the location of the tumour, various things can stop working. My tumour is in the area of the brain responsible for vision and I have a real problem seeing anything to the right of what I am looking at. It is irritating, but no more. Yet in front of that part are the areas responsible for motor control and speech. Damage there would give someone much more to contend with.

Coming back to read my e-mails was a great lift. Normally I read them during the week but this time I had been starved of Internet access for six days and came back to a great wodge of goodwill. They and the soothing words of the doctor have left me looking forward to the coming weeks. In a week's time I hope I will be able to report a trouble-free week spent exercising some new gadgets.

Thursday 14 November 2002

I feel as if I have spent the week with my jaws wide open like a roaring lion, except that my roars have been yawns. What little nausea I did experience from the chemotherapy was quickly brought under control by tablets I had been given. But the tiredness was inescapable. I found myself struggling to get up before midday, only to fall asleep again late in the afternoon. Then I felt better in the evenings and I could stay up until a normal bedtime.

My appetite has not disappeared but it has been poor. I struggle to finish two slices of toast and an apple for a late breakfast, and then I have no urge to eat until the evening. My weight is dropping, but then again at about 100 kilos or nearly 16 stone, I've got some to spare. About 8 kilos (roughly a stone) have disappeared overall, but I am sure most of that was due to my diet.

It is frustrating to be so useless at home. I have never been particularly well organised at domestic tasks, as anyone who has ever shared living space with me would testify. Over the past week I have even found pulling my weight impossible. But, having finished the chemotherapy tablets on Sunday, I'm starting to come out of the tunnel of tiredness.

Getting up in the morning is easier and I no longer feel like going straight back to bed as soon as I sit down to eat breakfast. And I am heartened that if the drugs are so powerful, they ought to be having some kind of effect on the tumour. I am heartened too to think that I can cope with whatever else I need in the way of treatment in the future. But spending so much time severely tired does leave me prey to darker thoughts and worries.

I am worried that we have already played the ace in the pack of tumour-killing cards, the radiotherapy. I asked my doctor whether I could have more radiotherapy if the tumour did not go away. He made it clear that my brain would not be able to stand such an aggressive dose of radiation ever again.

Way into the future, beyond the horizon I deal with at present, I could have a top-up dose of radiation if the tumour came back. If it came back sooner than that, it seems the weapons would be more chemotherapy and/or surgery.

I also had a minor panic about a lump I have had on the bottom of my foot for about a year. I suddenly thought of a friend, now fully recovered, who had a cancer which began with similar lumps, but on the neck. I started worrying that I had let something ride that should have been dealt with months ago.

My doctor was, however, unimpressed. And, as he himself pointed out, 'When your oncologist is unimpressed, you know it's good news.'

He said the lump was probably just an enlarged tendon.

My job now is to rest and to try to look after my immune system, which could take something of a battering from the chemotherapy. I am encouraged by the fact that while all those around me are coughing and sneezing with autumnal colds, I am still unscathed. Perhaps all the vitamins and healthy eating are doing some good.

Thursday 21 November 2002

Somehow I have just managed to steal a week away from my disease. For the last few days I have woken up to normal thoughts and I have spent those days doing relatively normal things. I do not know how I managed it, but it has been wonderful. It is as if someone had been pushing down on the top of my ribcage for the past three months and has now suddenly let go. I hope it lasts.

The fatigue from the chemotherapy seems to have gone completely, though now that I have a winter cold it is hard to be sure.

I know that I cannot ignore my condition entirely, but as an experiment, doing it for a week worked really well. It is hard to strike the right balance. Life is so much easier if I simply pretend there is nothing wrong with me.

'Live your own life, not the life of the tumour,' wrote another brain tumour patient in a support group magazine I saw recently, and I thought, 'What a great idea!' But at the same time there is still the urge to find out more about the disease and of course about experimental treatments. It would be awful to have missed out on something that could make a huge difference simply because I did not hear about it.

I worry that all this self-deception is going to rebound on me at some point, that it is somehow wrong to try to ignore what has happened. Still, it is not possible to get away from the subject of cancer for too long.

Right after enjoying an afternoon pizza in town – vegetarian, of course – I ran straight into a pack of the new breed of young, professional, street fund-raisers who wear smart bibs identifying the charity they are working for this week. This week they were collecting for a cancer research charity.

I thought that I was safe from the subject when I got home and sat down to begin the new Zadie Smith novel, only to find one of the principal characters diagnosed with a brain tumour in the prologue. Perhaps it is OK to forget the tumour as much as I can, because there are just so many things that will bring it to mind in any case.

For reasons which will have to wait until next week's diary, we've been unusually busy. But I did finally manage to find a t'ai chi teacher and I am looking forward to starting lessons at the beginning of next month.

The diet is going well and given that I feel so positive at the moment, perhaps the exercises will help stabilise things and keep me on a more even keel for the next round of chemotherapy. Despite the cold, I feel full of life and I want to keep things that way.

From: Nick, UK

I have a malignant brain tumour and, as I'm twenty-three years old, you can imagine this has come as a bit of a shock. Nevertheless, I'm not going to mope around feeling sorry for myself. Like you, I have taken an active role in my treatment. Although my radiotherapy does not begin until 4 December, I have been eating a diet high in flavanoids – the same as you're eating with all the greens and fresh fruit. Flavanoids are also in red wine (two glasses a day) and in green tea. My oncologist recommended this to me and I am definitely feeling healthier inside. I have no doubt in my mind that I will still be here in ten years and, by then, the drugs and treatment will have moved on. I'm putting all my faith into my doctors and all my concentration into getting better. Keep the positive attitude going; no doubt you will outlive many of your peers.

From: Chris, Northern Ireland

I had a breast tumour seven years ago, during which time I was a quivering wreck. However, that experience changed me forever. How did a materialistic and stressed-out young woman come to take enormous joy in the most simple things? Coming out of that tunnel was like being a child again. I can't imagine what sort of a cynical old git I'd grow into if I had been spared what I thought was awful at the time!

From: Adene, UK

I follow how you are doing and hope the tiredness eases – think of it as your body forcing you to let it concentrate its repair. Continue with the healthy diet, try liquidised drinks with fruit and milk – they take less energy to consume. Keep your mind fighting the cancer and yes, making people realise cancer exists and how it affects people is essential.

From: Tanya, England

I've been wanting to write to you to wish you well, but am worried that I might come across as negative among all the positive e-mails you have been receiving. I lost my mum early last year after a short battle with a rare and very aggressive cancer. She didn't really stand a chance but nonetheless she fought hard to stay positive and her only completely unselfish worry was how I'd cope without her. I wish you all the luck in the world, you truly deserve it.

From: Shirley Schofield, North Yorkshire

I am a nurse working mostly with palliative care patients. A consultant neurosurgeon has been talking to us about brain tumours and treatment and, feeling quite despondent at the end, suggested to us all that we should read your diary. I have sat here for near on an hour and have learnt more than any consultant can teach. I wish you success in your treatment and power to your pen/computer/gadgets.

6

Wedding Belles

I married my partner on Saturday.

We've had an eventful two-and-a-bit years together and just before I was diagnosed, we decided to get married and try to lead quieter lives together. I am very grateful that she decided to go ahead with the wedding.

I am a lucky man to enjoy her support and company and it was a pleasure to be able to tell her so in front of so many family and friends. I almost managed to get to the end of my speech without my voice cracking.

Our daughter had a whale of a time, grinning merrily at all the cameras and objecting only to our attempts to put flowers in her hair just before we walked up the aisle with her.

In all the conversations that followed the ceremony, the subject of my health came up mercifully rarely. Just as I did last week, I felt that I had managed to steal more time away from my condition.

My wife, as she is now, is much more of a private person than

I am. I think, however, that I would not be breaching my commitment to objectivity and to her privacy by saying that she looked absolutely fantastic.

Her wish for privacy is also the reason why I have not written more about how she is coping. I took the decision to write this diary together with her and I promised her then that I would respect her privacy in what I wrote. Now that the wedding is over, she needs to get on with her work and we still have family staying with us so we are not planning a honeymoon.

I feel like I would have a hard time coping with another trip even if we did have the time. I start another round of chemotherapy next week and, if the last time was anything to go by, I am in for another week of sleep.

After that we need to think about how and where to celebrate our daughter's first Christmas. Getting married is inevitably connected with looking forward and it is a tough thing to do when the future is such an unpredictable thing. There are no guarantees for any married couple but there are especially few certainties for us. But the wedding has reminded us of how much support and goodwill we have behind us.

It has also reminded me of how much I enjoy the company of my friends and family and how much of a lift that is when times are hard.

7

Reasons to Be Cheerful

Thursday 5 December 2002

I began my second course of chemotherapy just before sitting
down to write this. Just as last time, I have to take four very
serious-looking tablets each day for the next five days, together
with some tiny pills which will stop me feeling sick. Round three
is due to start on New Year's Day and round four – provisionally
the last – at the end of January.

During the gaps I hope that the drugs are mopping up any bits
of the tumour that did not succumb to the radiotherapy I had at
the beginning of my treatment. I will not know whether it has all
worked well until I have a brain scan sometime in the New Year.

Each chemotherapy round starts with a visit to my briskly
cheery cancer specialist, who checks that my immune system is
capable of withstanding another round of treatment. This time,
as always, he had words of encouragement, and even though I
know that I will be pretty tired by the weekend, I am in very good
spirits.

Beginning the second round has made me realise how much

time has gone by and how much I have been able to enjoy since I first had the shocking news at the end of August. I have had a struggle to remain positive, but there have been many things which have helped in that struggle. Last week's wedding was of course a huge highlight and I still find myself grinning inwardly about it, but seeing so much more of my family and so many good friends has also been a massive help.

People have reacted in different ways as I have told them about my tumour but the ones who have been the most help have been those who have quietly stepped up the frequency with which we meet and talk but have otherwise carried on as normal.

I have seen my daughter grow in confidence, learn to stand by herself and to speak her first words. Now we are making plans for her first Christmas.

And the great mercy I have enjoyed has been that I have suffered no symptoms from the tumour, other than the problems with my eyesight that I have had all year. I can walk around the city, go on the Underground, and feel like a normal person. I am so glad that all that has been possible and I am very optimistic about what I might be able to enjoy in the future.

This week I also finally managed to organise myself a t'ai chi lesson, though when the tutor arrived, it turned out that I am learning chi gong, which, in my ignorance, I think is a less physical and more health-oriented variant of the discipline.

I have a routine to do twice a day and though it is early days yet, I really feel it helps to make me relax and to clear my head. I have not been brave enough to do the routines outside yet, partly because of the rain, but principally for fear of what the neighbours might say.

I am going to try to keep up the exercises right through the week of tiredness and, in the meantime, before the chemotherapy side effects kick in properly, I am going to go out and enjoy the first of what I hope will be several Christmas parties.

Thursday 12 December 2002

The chemotherapy was much easier than last time.

Last time around I was struggling to stay awake only a couple of hours after I got out of bed. This time there has been fatigue, but nothing like as much. Perhaps last month I still had a hangover from the radiotherapy when I started the chemo.

Getting going in the morning is still a struggle but once I am up and out of the house I am fine. I only missed one day of my chi gong exercises. The trick seems to be making sure that I am going to see someone every day. If I only have a list of chores to work through then I put them off. The thing that continues to astonish me is how normal I feel.

It is testament to how effective my treatment has been so far. Whatever happens to me next, this part has been good. As I mentioned last week, it is so good to travel home on the Underground after having treatment. It is wonderful, even if there is nowhere to sit down. I feel in a way as if I am doing something I never expected to do.

I want to go back to work now. It is beginning to look as if I might manage a couple of half-days in the office before Christmas. That does not seem much, but it would be a start and it would give me something to improve upon when I get through round three in the New Year.

We have decided to spend our daughter's first Christmas in Germany with my wife's family. My parents will join us on Christmas Eve – the main day of celebration there.

It will be hectic, but our daughter's cousins will be there for her to enjoy it with, my sister-in-law and her husband are generous and welcoming hosts, and the chances of snow are better. Sticking to my diet is going to be a challenge.

The thought of this possibly being my last Christmas crosses my mind only now – as I am writing. An indication, perhaps, of how far my spirits have risen.

Last time I saw my doctor he had no specific news – there is none to be expected until I have my scan next year – but he did say things which gave me great encouragement. It is one thing to have decided for myself that things will turn out well but it is quite another to know that my doctor feels the same way.

I hope they do, for the both of us. I do not envy him his job. I am not sure how deliberate his management of how much I know about my tumour has been, but somehow it has been just right and his briskly confident manner has always made me feel better.

I do not know why some doctors seem to have this knack and others not. Obviously experience plays a big role but I have come across doctors who seemed very young but had completely mastered it.

I think it boils down to them being able to put themselves into the patient's shoes. Doctors need to be detached from the misery and distress involved in some of the diseases they treat. They also need their specialist vocabulary to be able to communicate with other doctors quickly. With the really scary diseases, some of that terminology is correspondingly scary.

But the doctors who have given me faith and hope have been those who have – for the time they were speaking to me – shed that detachment and vocabulary and become knowledgeable, confident but ordinary people.

For someone in my situation, faith and hope are priceless.

Wednesday 18 December 2002

Tomorrow is the day I intend going back to work.

It will not be much of a return, in that I will be in the office for two days before I go away for Christmas and then I will have more chemotherapy starting on 2 January.

Friday sees our team's Christmas lunch, so I do not expect a gruelling schedule. But, for me, it will be a statement of intent, another step on the road to leading as normal a life as possible.

Some time early next year I will find out if all the treatment I have been having has worked and whether real normality is going to be possible for any length of time. That is something I am usually optimistic about, but I cannot say I am looking forward to the day of the results very much.

I would have gone back to work a couple of days earlier, but I wanted to take my daughter to see her great-grandmothers, both of whom are ninety years old. That meant a trip home to Yorkshire, which is where I am writing this.

The healthier of my grandmothers was delighted to see her first great-grandchild and the two of them entertained each other happily. No one has told her about my diagnosis, only that I was in hospital, and it was awkward avoiding her occasional questions about my health. She lives in a home and her carers thought it better not to let her know. I did not argue.

As a person for whom reaching his forties is a great ambition, spending even less than an hour surrounded by people in their eighties and nineties provokes all kinds of odd thoughts. At first I thought it was great that I was unlikely to end up in a home in my nineties. Both sets of carers for my grandmothers do a great job and the homes are clean and comfortable but, all the same, I do not think I would be missing out on much.

Then I thought perhaps I will end up somewhere similar, just an awful lot earlier than them. I hope not.

But the thing that stuck in my mind was seeing photographs of my daughter and myself at the beginning of this year, just after she was born, and grieving for the unadulterated happiness of that time. In those days I had hair, but more importantly the expectation of spending decades with her and my wife.

There is no point wishing for miracles – I will be delighted if I hear next year that my treatment has gone well – but that expectation is now a dear hope. Living in hope is a very different way of life to living with expectations, however close to normality I come.

Christmas will see us in Germany with my wife's family and I am confident that the technology will co-operate to let me wish everyone who has given me so much support and encouragement since August a happy, peaceful and healthy New Year.

Wednesday 25 December 2002

Christmas here in Germany has been lovely. The white Christmas we were hoping for turned out to be grey, wet and unseasonably warm, but happily the proceedings were dominated by three excited children and a tableful of fantastic food and wine.

My parents flew over on Christmas Eve, just in time for the main celebrations here in the evening. There was a puppet show for the children, then presents for everyone, followed by dinner and conversation in alcoholically lubricated Anglo-German pidgin into the small hours.

Our little girl hooted and cackled her way through everything, taking great delight in unwrapping her presents, ignoring them and playing with the wrapping paper. It has been a great week, even if my diet has fallen by the wayside over the last couple of days.

Returning to work went well. I spent most of the first half-day saying hello to people and most of the second celebrating Christmas with my colleagues on the science and technology desks but I feel as if I achieved what I set out to do and put a toe in the water.

Once work was over on Friday I spent the weekend with a friend driving over to Germany, stopping overnight in Brussels. Again I found myself doing something I thought I would never do again when I was first told about my tumour.

We met up with a school-friend of mine who now lives in Brussels and walked the rain-soaked streets looking at the beautiful buildings for an hour before giving in to gluttony and the urge to taste the local beers.

I am writing this in the peace of the afternoon of Christmas Day and I had expected to feel more reflective.

I have just been through the most intense year of my life.

I became a father in January, was diagnosed with one of the most serious kinds of cancer there is in August, and got married in November.

I have experienced pure joy and pure terror. But I am afraid it has not left me with any pearls of wisdom to share.

I am quietly optimistic about what next year will bring and what I wish for myself and my family is what I wish all of you reading this, especially all the people who have given me such enormous support over the past few months.

It is what my wife said she would like as she visited me after my first night in hospital in August: 'Let us all have a quiet, uneventful year.'

There seems to be a war coming. I have my own little battle to fight. It would be marvellous if we were all to make it to next December unscathed.

From: Jana Mullerova, Czech Rep

When everything's fine there's nothing to talk about . . . I wish you no news next year, and all the years after, as boring and ordinary as possible.

From: David, Canada

I was particularly taken by your phrase: 'Living in hope is a very different way of life to living with expectations . . .' As a person living with a chronic/ terminal illness I understand this sentiment. You captured it so clearly and

44

concisely without any maudlin sensibility. In fact, I often think it's a blessing to live life this way – and more real.

From: Martin, Wales

I am so angry that this should happen to you – indeed to anyone. I wish you and your family the very best. It sounds like your daughter has a brave dad. I want her to be able to shout at you when she's a teenager. I'll be thinking of you this Christmas.

8

The Hunt for a Magic Bullet

Thursday 2 January 2003

The good news is that my hair is coming back.

Slowly, fine down like the hair on a baby's head is appearing on my forehead in the place where the last hairs fell out a couple of months ago. It looks like it will be a slow job. I am still bald as a coot around the back, where my scar is.

I have got used to my appearance – strangers still look twice at me and there is the occasional comment but I do not think people associate it with a brain tumour. Some, like the lads in the hotel bar the night before my wedding, think it is just an exotic haircut. Others, I think, assume I have a hair-loss disorder. I do not mind either way but I would love to look in the mirror and see my old face looking back at me.

Tomorrow I am due back at the hospital to start my third round of chemotherapy. I will have a blood test to see if my immune system is up to another round of treatment and then, all being well, a chat with the doctor and another with the pharmacist who gives out the pills.

Home in time for tea with friends from Turkey who are over for a fortnight. They are both specialists in treating cancer. I think they're brave to come and see me, knowing so much more about what I have and what is likely to happen to me than I do.

After the weekend I want to go back to the office while I am still taking the chemotherapy tablets but I do not know yet if I am going to be up to it. There are times when I feel woozy, or my head aches in the night or I feel for a split second like I am going to faint, and suddenly I panic because I cannot decide whether these are side effects of the treatment or a sudden turn for the worse. A friend once convinced me it was wrong to grieve over things that have not yet happened, but sometimes I just fail to take that particular medicine.

Dealing with panic is the part of my situation where I most need courage. I know that I will die one day, just like everybody else, but when I think of my own death, I think: 'Not now! Not now!' I have got too much left to do.

I am, as anyone who has read this diary in previous weeks will know, very, very grateful to my wife for her support, and to my family and friends. And the messages which appeared in response to what I wrote last week also gave me a great lift.

My colleagues at the BBC News website receive hundreds of e-mails sent in by readers of this diary, and forward them to me in batches, but often I do not see them until I write on a Wednesday. It is a great comfort to know that other cancer sufferers find it possible to fight their fight with courage and hope. And it is a privilege that I have such a public forum for this diary and as a result am part of the hopes and wishes of people I have never met.

Monday 13 January 2003

It is very strange to be writing this diary from my desk in the office for the first time. I took the last chemotherapy tablets of this current round on Monday and I am still pretty groggy – sleepy, forgetful and easily distracted.

The feeling reminds me of when I used to work nights. After the first night I would be sitting in my normal surroundings but with the distinct feeling that something was missing. I am clearly not firing on all cylinders and if someone ran through the office with no clothes on, it would take me about five minutes to notice. But it feels good to be at work and trying to return to some kind of normality.

I arrive late and leave early, so the days are very short, but at least I am here. Time and time again I am struck by how surreal the whole thing is. I have one of the most dangerous cancers around, yet here I am writing and talking about stories we will cover later in the year.

Why do I feel so well if I have such a serious condition? It seems wrong to question my good fortune, but it does seem as if my only immediate problems are ones which are a result of the treatment rather than the disease.

Introspection and paranoia are a real problem. Every time I forget something, I ask myself whether I would have forgotten it a year ago. One of the areas of the brain which is responsible for language is in front of where my tumour is and so every time I stumble over words, say the wrong word or even get mixed up between English and German at home, I try to think whether I have always slipped up so often or whether it has got worse.

I regularly worry that I am putting on a great show of normality for myself and the rest of the world, as if I was trying to trick the tumour into believing that I'm fine. I can hear a voice telling me to snap out of it, get on with life and not be such a bloody whingeing fool, but that does not stop the worries – it just means I feel daft for having them.

When I saw the doctor this time, it was only briefly, and he told me that the scan to see if my treatment has worked will be at the beginning of March. It is hard to keep track, but it does seem as if he has constantly been putting it back.

I have managed to convince myself that he has been delaying because he has had no cause for concern so far. My chances of a reasonable period of remission seem fairly good and the date is too far off to start worrying about yet. But when the time comes, it's not going to be easy to go and have the scan.

Back to the present – the highlight of the week has been our little girl's first encounter with snow. Quite sensibly she thinks it is very nice to look at, hooting with enthusiasm from the window at the white-dusted back garden, but not much fun to be out in on your way to nursery.

Thursday 16 January 2003

We have just been celebrating my daughter's first birthday with banana cake, a candle and a glittery hat. She is too young, of course, to realise the significance of the occasion, but she had a great time with the rest of the kids at the nursery, stuffing handfuls of cake into her mouth without a thought for cutlery or convention, yet presiding regally over the afternoon tea table.

All three of us are fighting a winter cold which she brought home one day last week, but it has not stopped us thoroughly enjoying the day. It was wonderful to see her having fun and to have a happy occasion on which to look back at a chaotic and eventful year. I never expected life to be like this, with joy and mortal fear so close together.

Someone who has been living with cancer much longer than me e-mailed last week with an observation that really helped. I hope she doesn't mind me paraphrasing what she said, but the core of it was that as you make progress, you stop counting the 'lasts' and start counting the 'firsts'.

She was referring to the temptation that strikes every time there is a Christmas, birthday or other chronological event to think: 'This could be my last.' Marking the firsts is a much better idea. Soon I hope to be celebrating my first week after ending my treatment.

My little girl stands on her own two feet now and I want to see her first unaided steps. And, most of all, I want to understand what she is saying.

She talks incessantly, but all I can make out is: 'Bye bye', 'Papa' (which refers mostly to me but often to the nearest person, male or female) and 'Apple' (which refers to a range of edible substances). It will be great when we achieve our first two-way conversation.

Slowly life feels as if it is expanding into a medium-term possibility. It is not something I can count on, of course – the scan at the end of February could pull the rug from under me – but I have begun to lose the feeling that I should not tempt fate by thinking beyond the end of the treatment.

I hope that is not too rash.

Thursday 23 January 2003

It has been a good week. In theory, I should find it harder than normal to fight off infections because chemotherapy not only attacks cancer cells; it also has an effect on the immune system. But I shook off the cold that came on at the end of last week in a couple of days. Perhaps all the vitamin supplements I take are doing some good. Normally I would have needed at least a week to feel normal again.

I am getting up earlier and earlier, staying awake longer and even managed a couple of pints and a curry one night this week – another notch on the yardstick of normality. I think the chi gong might have something to do with my improving strength.

I really let it go over Christmas and New Year but, having sheepishly confessed this to my instructor, I have managed my exercises virtually every day since. My legs ache from all the standing with knees unlocked but I am much more relaxed and feel that I am walking and standing upright for once.

Our little girl has been in a great mood since her birthday and is experimenting unsuccessfully with taking her first steps. Our ancestors evolved into bipeds to free their hands to use tools but so far the point is lost on her. She can reach a fair old speed on all fours even with a toy or remote control in hand.

She was less than impressed when I gave her her first haircut. Two snips removed enough of her fringe for her to see out again, but she resisted with the vigour she usually reserves for attempts to wipe her runny nose.

At work I have been researching a special section to mark the fiftieth anniversary of the publication of the structure of DNA. When James Watson and Francis Crick published details of the now iconic double helix in April 1953, it took years for their work to become fully appreciated. But in time, scientists have uncovered a world of knowledge about what goes wrong in DNA to give some people conditions such as cancer, Alzheimer's disease, Huntington's chorea, cystic fibrosis, diabetes or early heart problems.

The human genome project's completion of its first draft in 2000 was more evidence of the huge progress scientists have made in understanding what makes humans what they are and what makes them ill. The galling thing, though, for someone in my position is how little of this knowledge seems to have been turned into cures.

I live with a researcher and I understand why the pace of research has to be so painstakingly slow. I believe the cures will come and I have great hopes that progress will be made on dealing with my type of tumour in the next few years. But it is hard to escape the feeling that for most diseases that result from dodgy DNA, the cures people might have hoped for in 1953 are still not here.

Our understanding of them has become far more sophisticated. We can test for them and in some cases we have a much better idea of how people will do as they live with the disease. But in most cases, the magic bullets we once hoped for are still on the armourer's test bench.

From: Colby Jarvis, England

My dad has been diagnosed with lung cancer and the cancer centres can be so daunting and people are so quiet; without meaning to be it becomes a depressing environment. We should encourage people to support each other more and this is what your column is doing. While people's e-mails support you, you in turn are supporting us.

From: Debbie Robertson, UK

I have often been inspired by your forthrightness. I sense a change in your approach to your illness – all I can say is don't give up hope. I was a neurosurgical nurse for many years and have seen this so often. Cherish what you have now and in your future, and always appreciate, communicate with, and love those who are near to you. I wish you nothing but good times.

From: Michael, Netherlands

Good to hear you are back at work and getting back into some semblance of normality (if by normal, you mean staring at a screen like the rest of us). Try not to worry about stumbling over your words. We all do it from time to time and you've said that you're tired too so it's bound to happen. If you focus on it, you'll make it worse by stressing yourself. Have you ever crept around the house to avoid waking the children? That's the most likely time for you to drop a saucepan on the floor or accidentally slam a door.

From: Eunice Young, N. Ireland

Do you realise just how much good you have done by writing this diary? My husband has just been diagnosed with an incurable brain tumour and reading your column every week lets us know roughly what to expect. Now he has a positive attitude and can't wait to get his first zap of radiotherapy at the end of this month. Keep up the good work, as it's working wonders for everyone.

From: Catherine, UK

Thanks for reminding my why I'm in science. Many times during the last eighteen months of my biochemistry Ph.D.

I've cursed my choice of career path, as progress is painstakingly slow. It's often hard to see how your piece fits into the jigsaw. Keep believing in the magic bullet but with your positive attitude something tells me you won't need it.

From: Mel Morris, UK

I have a degenerative condition which affects my joints. I keep saying: 'Did I always stumble over kerbs that big or is that new?' But don't feel daft – I'm sure I won't be the only one to empathise unless I'm daft too. I'm glad to hear you are back at work; normality is good for the psyche if nothing else.

9

Layers of Normality

'Congratulations!' said my doctor, as we shook hands and I left his consulting room. I have just picked up the tablets for my last round of chemotherapy.

On Sunday I will have finished five-and-a-half months of treatment – six weeks of radiotherapy followed by four months of chemo – all of it, thankfully, as an outpatient.

When we started my treatment my oncologist said that I was a young man with everything to fight for and that he would 'throw the book' at the tumour. Now that we have finished hurling medical literature about, I have dates in my diary in early March for a brain scan which will tell us where it landed.

Smack bang on top of the tumour, I hope.

I know now what it means to be cautiously optimistic. I am not superstitious but at the same time making plans as far ahead as summer feels like tempting fate. I feel and look fit and well and I am looking forward to February – a whole month without medical appointments.

I want to fly to Hong Kong, where my brother lives, to meet my first and only nephew, whom I have only seen in photos. And I want to hatch plans for one or two less grand weekend trips closer to home. It seems to work if I take things a month at a time. I planned nothing for February and put off anyone who tried to pin me down for anything until I saw the doctor today. Now February feels like a present I have been given, a big chunk of time not spoken for, like a lawn with fresh snow.

In the past I have said thank you for all the e-mails of support I have had but I am particularly moved to say thank you again this week. I have had a sudden spate of interviews to do and I am always asked what makes me write this diary. Sometimes I ask myself the same question, but it is always answered when I read e-mails saying 'thanks for reminding me why I'm in science' or from someone saying it has helped them in the way they care for patients.

Just after I was diagnosed in August, my wife said to me that, whatever happened, we should try to make something positive out of what was happening to me. I was and am deeply grateful to her for everything she said and did for me in those black and desperate days and if I have managed to do as she suggested in this diary then I am very happy.

Thursday 6 February 2003

My treatment's over, even though it doesn't quite feel like it yet. I finished the last of the chemotherapy tablets on Sunday and I have been pretty tired ever since. But if the last three months are anything to go by, I should feel better by the weekend. I will have to, because by the time this is published I will be landing in Hong Kong.

The only drugs I am taking now are very mild, intended to prevent the epileptic fits which sometimes affect people with brain tumours. But every day I still take a whole handful of vitamin supplements which are meant for those with problems of the immune system.

People keep telling me how well I look. I feel it, too.

Half of me feels like rushing ahead to make plans and the other half feels like taking the doctor's advice and waiting until the scan results in early March. There is plenty to be getting on with right now, though. Our little girl managed her first steps at the weekend, or at least the first ones either of us was there to witness. I am sure she has been practising at her nursery.

She slowly and carefully tottered six steps across her bedroom floor towards me before giving up and sitting down again. She can tell that I am especially proud of her and has now learnt to say 'two' whenever I hold up a finger and say 'one'. A big part of me does not want to go away to Hong Kong at all, because it means not seeing her for six days.

I have become a lot more careful about how I spend my time and without totally giving up on a social life, I try to spend as much of it as possible at home with her and her mother.

Dealing with my decades-old computer addiction can be tricky, though. We first had a computer at home when I was about fifteen and ever since then I have been utterly fascinated with the little worlds inside them. I must have spent years of my life by taking computers apart, putting them back together, reconfiguring them and trying to connect them together in various ways.

Without all that tinkering, I would not have the job I have today, but I can quite understand that most people would view it as a waste of time. I made a promise to myself after I was diagnosed not to buy any more computer games and especially not to buy a games console. If life does turn out to be too short for me, then I do not want my final achievement to be a high score on Halo.

I do wish I could figure out file-sharing between my Mac and my PC, though.

Thursday 13 February 2003

Sitting in a quayside bar enjoying the view of Hong Kong Island in the distance and watching the ferries come and go, I had to remind myself who and what I was. I never manage a whole day without thinking about my condition, but I was close to it during the time I was away.

The long weekend with my brother and his new family was great fun and I was really pleased to see my nephew at last. But the trip made me even more aware of how jarring it can be to slip in and out of normality.

I find myself seduced into thinking far into the future, about where my daughter might go to school, about whether we should live in Germany or England, and then, all of a sudden, I remember how serious my condition is and how little I can count on in the future. It is as if I can put on my old life like a comfortable old coat, relax into it, but then suddenly have someone come to take it away again.

It is now almost six months since my confidence in the future was shattered by my diagnosis. I am getting much better at dealing with the emotional consequences, but it is still hard work.

Having little to deal with on the physical side right now makes the job easier, but I am having trouble knowing how far forward I should allow myself to look. Living life a month at a time is manageable.

But real life is not like that. My wife and I both travel with our jobs and we have trips we need to plan in March and June. Is it OK to plan a work trip in June? I do not know. There is no rule book for my situation.

People have said to me that making plans for the future is part of life and that I should go ahead and make them. I can see their logic and I know they are right, but I am scared. I am afraid of suffering terrible disappointment.

It seems easier to work with low expectations and celebrate

everything that does go well than start to count on too many things. I am physically fit and have every reason to be optimistic about what I will hear next month but I still feel uncomfortable thinking beyond then. Seizing the day, or the month, even, seems fine to me but seizing the year seems like too much to take all at once.

Life right now is wonderful. I just want to slow time down and let it trickle past.

Thursday 20 February 2003

This week's challenge is chickenpox. Our little girl was sent home from nursery on Monday with a number of interesting-looking spots, confirmed by the doctor that afternoon as chickenpox. She is bright and breezy and utterly unconcerned – we have not reached the scratching phase yet – so I am not too worried about her, but I am worried she might infect me.

I had chickenpox as a child but apparently there is still the danger that I might contract shingles, caused, I think, by the same virus. So until she gets better, I am taking antiviral tablets four times a day on top of the anti-epilepsy drugs I already have and my daily vitamin cocktail.

Staying at home to look after her the last two days has meant me seeing a lot more of her than I usually do. It has been lovely to see her practise her walking, and to enjoy the colourful spectacle of her mealtimes, but it comes at a time when I am finding it tough to find the energy not to get too preoccupied with my forthcoming scan. I don't think there's any specific reason not to be optimistic about the results but it is still preying on my mind.

Now is a very strange time. At first, when I was diagnosed, I was in a state of shock, but after that I was surprised at how easily I found it to accept that life was suddenly going to be very, very different.

I had treatment to worry about and get on with, and this diary to write. Dealing with cancer became my job. But now the chunks of normality that I have had have started me thinking about what it would be like if I did not have to worry about the tumour any more, if I could suddenly stop living in the here and now and make long-term plans.

That is inconceivable, for the time being.

It is very difficult to know what to do for the best.

Whatever happens, I want to be prepared.

I want to have the emotional strength to complete whatever I have to do with dignity, to rejoice if I have reason to and, if not, to be strong and to leave everyone with positive memories if I do have to make an unscheduled exit. The trouble is that there just seems to be no way of preparing myself. I try to steer a steady course between total denial of what is happening to me and excessive pessimism, but I end up swerving all over the place.

There is no handbook for how to do this right and if there was, I would probably be too much of a coward to read it. I desperately want to win this fight, to see more walking and more messy lunchtimes.

I hope that I learn how along the way.

Thursday 27 February 2003

It has been a busy week and busy has meant less time to worry. Our daughter's chickenpox disappeared almost as quickly as it appeared. Either she has a superhuman immune system or, more likely, she had a really mild dose. It is a harmless enough infection for most children, but nevertheless I am very glad to see her back to normal. She did look very funny covered in calamine lotion, though.

Her rapid recovery has meant that I am back at work, where I am happy to find myself working on three different things at once and, I hope, not making too big a hash of any of them.

Putting back on the layers of normality and finding that they are comfortable and still fit is a really good feeling.

When I was first diagnosed, I was catapulted forwards in my life to a position where I thought my life was almost over, as if I had become an old man overnight. Now I have no particular evidence that this has changed except for the fact that I continue to feel strong and well.

I have decided to try to tackle all the anxiety about my scan by being more willing to make plans and get back into what was my normal life. Looking after our daughter last week was hard work but great fun at times. Then going back to work I found myself caught up in thinking about what I am working on and I realised that these are the things I want to do. I was doing them before because I wanted to, so there is no reason to stop now.

I will always have scans and tests to face so I think that I should try not to let the worry make me put things on hold. Having things on hold means having time to dwell on my worries and that is what allows them to grow.

The other thing that has made me less miserable about the scan is realising that even if things went really badly and I was not around for much longer, I would be leaving at a happy time. I spent a very long time looking for the kind of relationship I now have with my wife. When our little girl joined us, I could not – and still cannot – think of anything that I would ever want to change.

Of course it would be a tragedy if I had to leave them but I feel strong enough to hope that I will not have to just yet. All this introspection has been uncomfortable and tiring, not just for me, but I hope now that I can be a better father, colleague and husband as a result.

From: An admirer, England

I can well understand your unwillingness
to spend as much time playing on the
computer, but I hope you don't feel that
because you are a survivor of a terrible
illness, that you have to fill the rest
of your life with virtue? Why not buy
some more computer games?! Allow yourself
some little indulgences! Life is a gift
which you are enjoying and nothing you
can do can take back the past.
Personally, I am amazed by my husband's
pleasure at playing computer games but he
enjoys it! Enjoy your daughter, enjoy
your wife but also, enjoy yourself! Good
luck with 'Halo' (whatever that is).

From: Deborah, UK

However bad the problem is it never seems
so scary when you know that others have
gone through the same thing. You are
doing a lot of people a lot of good by
sharing your experiences. Some time ago,
over several years, I suffered from
multiple benign breast cysts and other
lumps. I had medical insurance so as each
new lump appeared I would make an
appointment to see the specialist at a
local private hospital. Each time I would
wait in the deep-pile-carpeted waiting-
room, anxiously watching the other
patients sitting there looking so
composed in their smart clothes reading

their posh newspapers (how they could
read newspapers if they were feeling as
anxious as I was I could never
understand), and talking in hushed tones.
Eventually I reached the outpatient limit
on my insurance and became an NHS
patient. I now found myself waiting in
tatty, overcrowded waiting-rooms with
ordinary - i.e. unintimidating - women -
who would *talk* to me! It made *such* a
difference. I had been apprehensive about
using NHS facilities but having now made
the switch I wouldn't go back to those
hushed tones and deep-pile carpets. Put
me in a crowd of women, all in the same
boat, and I am a lot happier. You are
doing an excellent one-man job of
providing waiting-room support and
camaraderie for I guess thousands of
patients across the world.

From: Andrew Moody, UK

What strikes me is how we are happy in
our ignorance of what the future holds
for us. Yet we are all lucky - first in
not having to face your current trial and
second in having the chance to change our
priorities without such a terrifying
prompt. Unfortunately, I fear we will be
moved by your experience but still fail
to embrace what is really important.

From: Tracey, USA

I've had four brain tumours. I've been
dealing with this round for about
eighteen months . . . the first was removed
in 1991. I had my MRI scan last Sunday
and now am waiting to hear the results.
There is always worry and fear, but this
time some symptoms have come back, and
I'm expecting to hear I need surgery . . .
even more stress. I'm not working, but I
take college classes to keep busy. I tend
to mark the time by going from one
semester to another . . . 'If I can just
finish this semester I'll be OK.' It's
hard to think further ahead than that, so
I know what you mean about being hesitant
to make plans for the future. I talk
about the future in theory but I have no
idea if I will actually be here for it.
I'm just thirty-three, and don't have any
kids, although I would love to have some.
I can't help wondering if it would be
fair. I don't really know what the answer
is. Good luck - enjoy this time of joy
in your life, and encourage those around
you to realise their own.

From: Zalie, USA

I have two acquaintances each diagnosed
with the most aggressive form of brain
tumour. They're not completely well, but
they are living actively and
productively. The one thing they seem to

have in common is an apparently total rejection of statistics. One of them has tried alternative treatments. The other just forges ahead. I love their spirit and hope that you will not let superstitious fear of tempting fate deprive you of the same sort of mind-over-matter strength.

10

Crunch Time

Thursday 6 March 2003

I had a brain scan on Monday to see whether all the treatment I have had over the last six months has worked. I have not got the results yet but I will have soon. It is a very nervous time, but I am trying to stay busy and positive, telling myself that I am feeling fit and that that has to be a good sign.

The scan itself was short and sweet. It was an MRI (magnetic resonance imaging) scan, similar to the one I had when I was diagnosed last year. MRI scanners work by subjecting the body to huge magnetic fields. Different tissues in the body respond slightly differently to magnetic fields because they are made of slightly different percentages of the basic elements. These varying responses allow the scanner to build up a picture of what is inside the body in a far more detailed way than an X-ray.

Because the machine uses such powerful magnetic fields, you have to be sure that you have no metal either on or in your body. I managed to get away with the couple of gold inlays I have in my teeth but apparently even metal dust in the eye from an industrial accident would be enough to cause problems.

The whole scan took less than twenty minutes. The scanner is a huge cylindrical thing with a person-sized tunnel through it into which the patient slots. I lay down on my back on a trolley and the radiographers slotted the top half of my body into the machine. I can imagine that people who suffer from claustrophobia might find it unsettling, but thankfully I do not fall into that category.

This particular scanner had a mirror immediately in front of my eyes which worked like a periscope to let me see down past my feet to watch the radiographers moving around in the control room. I felt more comfortable with my eyes shut and might have happily nodded off had the machine not been such a noisy thing.

As it lets loose the various pulses it needs to build up a full picture, it makes a hammering sound – not deafening but nevertheless fairly distracting.

Towards the end of the scan a radiographer came to inject me with what he described as 'contrast'. This substance makes the blood flow in the body show up better on the scan. As tumours grow, they need their own blood supplies and have a way of making the body grow new arteries to supply them. So it is important for doctors to have a clear idea of where blood is going in the area around the tumour.

When I think about how important the results of this scan are, I freeze with fear. Suppressing that fear costs a lot of energy and it is making me tired. But very soon I will have the results and will then at least know a bit more about what is to come.

Friday 7 March 2003

'It's good news,' said my doctor, before my wife and I had even sat down in his office. We had gone to receive the results of the first brain scan I have had since my initial diagnosis.

I sank into a chair in relief, held my wife's hand and waited for him to explain.

He gave us the best news possible, that my tumour has responded well to my treatment and has shrunk. I will have another brain scan in six months and in the meantime I do not need any more treatment.

'Go out and enjoy your life,' he said.

He showed us the scan films but I could not bear to look, so my wife did for me. The inside of my head apparently still does not look too pretty and it never will. Even if the tumour never regrows it will still be there in some form. And tumours of the kind I have are very likely to come back.

'You know the stats as well as I do,' my doctor said. The tumour is not bound to regrow but it probably will. If it does then I will need more treatment and will have another fight on my hands.

But that is a worry for the future. The far future, as far as I am concerned right now. What I have been given now is six months during which I have no real reason to worry about anything, plus the prospect of still being around in what he called 'the years to come'.

Six months is a huge chunk of time – the same length of time we have been dealing with this cancer so far. I have every reason to believe that I will be around for another Christmas, for our little girl's second birthday, for all the things I have not dared seriously to contemplate.

I am very grateful to all the people who have helped me win the first round of the fight and to become a cancer survivor.

My GP did the right thing and got me into hospital quickly. The neurosurgeons were quick with their diagnosis and the nursing staff kept me comfortable in the meantime. My cancer specialist is a man with a real gift for sustaining hope and quite clearly knows his medical onions. Therapeutic radiographers designed and administered the radiotherapy which has been the main weapon in pushing back the tumour. Staff at the hospital looked after me during chemotherapy and my scan.

My wife has given me strength and support at every turn and our daughter has been an inspiration. The rest of my family have helped me hold my life together with much encouragement and practical help. Countless friends have helped to remind me how lucky I am and what I have to stay around for.

My editors and colleagues at the BBC have made travelling the road back to work a pleasure. And the readers of this diary have on many occasions provided faith and hope to get through another difficult day.

Thank you, all of you.

Thursday 13 March 2003

Last week's scan result has given me my life back, for the time being at least.

By the time that this is published, I will be in Germany reporting on the world's biggest IT fair, CeBIT 2003. Last time I was on a reporting trip was six weeks before my diagnosis.

At the weekend we started making holiday plans: to see my wife's family in Germany at Easter and then go to a friend's wedding in France in May. I want to continue writing my diary. Round one has gone to me, but I haven't won the fight by any stretch of the imagination. So from now on, as long as there is any interest, I will be writing every month instead of every week.

Lots of people have e-mailed me with suggestions about how I can look after myself better. I am going to try to spend more time on my chi gong and I also want to tighten up on my diet.

We have not heard about any large-scale scientific experiments concerning the effects of nutrition on cancer therapy, but I am working on the assumption that eating better cannot do me any harm and might do a whole lot of good. I have been told about a centre in the USA which combines conventional cancer treatment with dietary improvements and I am trying to find out if there is anything similar in the UK. The diet the US people propose sounds fairly strict but by no means weird; more or less a detox diet. Despite all my treatment, I am still overweight, so I am sure it will help in that respect if nothing else.

Over the six months I've been writing, I've heard from so many people who are either fighting cancer themselves or have someone very close to them who is. It is dreadful that we still have not wiped out such a destructive disease and I wish the very best of luck to all of those people who are trying bit by bit to eliminate it. And I hope that my good fortune shows that even with some of the most serious and deadly cancers, victories are possible.

From: Ricky Price, Scotland

I leapt out of my chair as if Dundee United had scored a goal in the Cup Final when I read this! I'm massively pleased for you and your family, Ivan - I hope you never have to go through all this again, and you've got my best wishes in everything you want to do. All the best, mate!

From: Rob, England

BACK OF THE NET!! Blinding news!

From: Mal Gray, Wales

Keep looking forward - it's the only way to travel.

From: Amy, UK

I know you're going to have a lot of e-mails exactly like this one, but I don't really care. I just want to let you know how very, very pleased I am for you, the relief must be exquisite. Have a lovely day.

From: Julie, UK

How fantastic for you all! Like many I held my breath as I read the latest news and felt absolute relief for you and your family - well done the NHS for spurring you on with their care and knowledge. Enjoy!

From: Liz Lewis, England

I work as a community nurse in London on night duty and have been following your diary with interest. Tonight it was with tears in my eyes as normally we nurses in the community only get to hear about the worst cases - to hear that sometimes people do beat the odds provides us all with hope and I wish you good health for as long as possible.

From: Klaus, Los Angeles

Makes us all wonder if we really live our lives to the fullest, live every day as if our days were numbered. Most of all let's not sweat about the small stuff. It's courage and attitude that keeps us healthy, I believe, so given your spirit and strength you'll have a bright and long, long future ahead of you!

Reflection – Simon Marshall

For a long time, I resisted sending in any comments to the diary, as I didn't think I would have anything really useful to say. But in the end I did write – I'm not sure why, I think it must have been partly for my own good.

My wife and I had our son James in June 2001. In his first few months, he seemed to be a big child, and at times seemed a bit lazy. He just didn't do natural things; he didn't bear weight on his feet, or respond well to toys, for instance. He would have a few spurts of energy and then go lazy again. We also noticed his eyes were wobbling a lot, so we took him to the GP and he was referred to have an MRI scan.

That very night, just a few hours after the scan, the three of us were rushed to Newcastle General Hospital, about an hour's drive away. It was 20 December, but suddenly things like Christmas didn't seem so important. They had found a tumour, an optic glioma, which was growing along the optic nerve and backwards into the brain. They did a biopsy on his tumour on Christmas Eve – we spent Christmas Day itself standing watching him in intensive care – this little boy who wasn't even a year old.

They decided to give James chemotherapy – he was too young to be able to have radiotherapy. He had one-hour sessions every week for ten weeks, and then monthly sessions for a year. The tumour stopped growing for a few months, but when it started again, they tried another form of chemotherapy, which was unsuccessful. The third kind they tried was being pioneered by an Italian doctor who was having remarkable results – every child in his test was showing signs of remission. After six or seven sessions, scans showed James's tumour had shrunk – we had to be careful not to get too carried away – but the tumour was now half the size it had been.

I think the parent of anyone who has cancer, but particularly someone very young, will share some of our feelings. I remember saying at first that this was impossible, it just wasn't happening. I remember – it's dreadful to confess it – that I felt I almost wanted to take him back to the shop and get one that worked properly. As a parent that's a horrible thing to think about. Almost a feeling of having created something that you now don't want. We asked the consultant if we had done anything wrong. Was there something about us that had made James have this cancer? All he could say was that we hadn't done anything wrong, and that we had just been unlucky.

That was so hard to take – if we had done something wrong then we could at least have warned other people. In fact if we did ever see a pregnant woman smoking or drinking, we wanted to go up to her and say that she could do something to prevent harming her child – we hadn't had that opportunity. As a parent, you would do anything – absolutely anything – to take away your child's suffering. Many's the time that Rachael and I said we would have willingly have James's cancer for him.

But there's no answer, and there are no solutions. We learnt to shut those feelings off and get on with day-to-day life. For three years now, our whole lives have revolved around James's health. When someone has chemotherapy, they are very susceptible to infections, and often James would have to be rushed back into Newcastle General where Rachael would stay with him for a week. Of course she's had to give up her job, because everything has become so unpredictable for us.

But James has grown into a fantastic little boy. We absolutely adore him. He's developing, but we think he's about a year behind where he would otherwise have been. He can say 'yes' and 'no', but has trouble pronouncing consonants. He is learning to communicate with a form of the Makaton sign language. At the moment he's learning to shout – and the number of people who comment on what a happy child he is, it's amazing. I still dream of doing those things with him that every father probably wishes to do – like kicking a ball in the park or going to the match – but we'll have to see about that.

The older he gets now, the greater the chance of him being able to have radiotherapy should the tumour grow back. But his consultant says his aim is to help James have a normal, full life. He says he wants him to be sitting as an 80-year-old in the pub, having a pint, chatting about how he had cancer as a boy. Ten years ago they might not have been able to do that for him, but now he's in with a chance.

11

My Summer of Love

Tuesday 15 April 2003

Only five weeks have passed since I had the good news that my tumour had shrunk but it is already difficult to make myself think about it. Now that it is no longer an immediate threat to my life, I have got on with things as my doctor said I should. We have been planning holidays and thinking about the future.

Not long after I had my brain scan result I went to see another specialist for an informal chat and his words were even more reassuring. He seemed confident that I would be around in five years' time and that treatments would have improved by then.

I was delighted to hear his opinion. The thing that gave me most confidence was to hear him say that if he divided all the patients with my type and grade of tumour into groups according to how well he expected them to do, I would be in the very top group.

It is extremely unlikely that my tumour will not come back to trouble me again – that is in the nature of my type of tumour –

but I have a good chance of it being years from now. And there will still be options in terms of how to deal with it then. My daughter is speaking and walking now. I can watch her and play with her without the terrible feeling I had before that this might all be over soon.

What I have to do is to try to remember the lessons the last seven months have taught me. I can put things in my diary for next month without feeling like I am tempting fate. And I have seen my name on stories on the front page of our website again but now the stories are nothing to do with cancer. That is a good feeling.

Living with so much low-level but relentless fear has been very tiring. Looking back, I think that much of the fatigue I had during radiotherapy and chemotherapy was a side effect not of the treatment but of the fear. And even today there are days when it is a battle to get going because all that I want to do is be in what feels like the safest place on Earth: asleep.

But life is good and it is so much easier now. What I have to do, besides hauling myself out of bed at a reasonable time each day, is to try to remember the lessons the last seven months have taught me and not to waste precious time.

Wednesday 14 May 2003

Time has begun to pass at its normal slightly alarming rate again. Before I had the good news from my scan in March the time crept by and I was grateful for the fact. Now it is zooming by, perhaps because I am enjoying my life again. I liked it before I was ill and I like it even more now.

But still there are times when the panic comes back and I silently brace myself for a premature return of the tumour. There was some apparent good news on the research front this month when a team in the USA announced that they had had good results testing a new technique to kill my type of tumour in rats.

They use a modified form of the common cold virus to attack the cancer cells in the brain.

Other teams, including some in the UK, are using similar techniques, including one which uses the diphtheria toxin. With all of them the idea is to attach some kind of nasty poison to something which homes in on the tumour cells and not the normal healthy cells.

It is a tricky thing to get right and there is plenty of potential for doing serious damage to the brain if things go wrong. At the moment these therapies all involve injections directly into the tumour, which, of course, means more brain surgery. Some of these approaches have progressed beyond animal trials to trials on human patients but none seem reliable enough to be ready for approval yet.

Reading about this kind of research is hard. It is fantastic that there are people who are working right now to find ways not just to manage but also to completely eradicate tumours like mine.

But the progress is necessarily slow, the testing periods long and who knows if and when these revolutionary new therapies will be available? And the press releases I read which describe these steps forward never fail to mention that what I have is considered 'the deadliest form of brain tumour'.

Every time I read something like that, and every time I realise that I am having trouble reading something because of the damage the tumour caused to my eyesight, I remember what has happened to me. I have built up a fragile pyramid of hopes and rationalisations to keep me going and, at these moments, it wobbles precariously. I don't suppose that will ever change.

Monday 16 June 2003

Three months have passed now since I had the good news that the first phase of treatment of my tumour had worked. Last year, when I was diagnosed, I did not realise it fully, but it was by no means certain that I would see another birthday.

So, just now as I celebrated my thirty-sixth, I had more reason than most people to celebrate.

But it is hard to celebrate whole-heartedly when the future is so uncertain. The rate of relapse for people who have what I have is terrifyingly high. And however many times I remind myself that statistics apply to groups, not individuals, and that as a young(ish) man with no major symptoms I have the best possible chance, I still find the battle against anxiety a difficult one.

So I have decided to spend two days at a centre which specialises in complementary treatment for cancer and a holistic approach to health. I have always had the strong feeling that besides all the treatment I have had, there ought to be something I could do to help myself.

I am already doing some of the things which the centre's literature describes. I am trying to keep up with my chi gong exercises to keep me strong and relaxed, I take a cocktail of vitamins every day and most of the time, birthdays and holidays notwithstanding, I stick to a diet free from meat, egg and dairy products. But I am hoping that the stay at the holistic centre will help me pull it all together and above all get to grips with the fear.

Whether I make it to see my little girl turn eighteen or whether the statistics catch up with me long before then, I do not want to spend the rest of my life curling up in bed in fear. It is important for my survival that I stay positive and it is crucial to the people close to me, too.

I am writing my diary every month now, so I hope that next month I will be singing the praises of self-help.

Wednesday 16 July 2003

I wanted to know as little as possible about my tumour when I was first diagnosed. I was so scared that I thought that whatever

I might learn would inevitably be worse than I already imagined things to be. All I wanted to know was that something could be done for me and all I wanted to do was get the treatment started.

But of course it is not possible to live a life of ignorance. Facts trickle out and by now, over ten months later, treatment complete and apparently in remission, I know the truth. Doctors do not try to cure tumours like mine because it is not possible using today's treatments. Instead they manage them, seeking to prolong life as long as possible and maintain as high a quality of life as possible.

They use radiotherapy, chemotherapy and surgery to keep the tumour at bay for as long as they can. Despite these efforts, half of all patients with my diagnosis die within the first year of their diagnosis. I am told that the number who make it to five years is less than one in ten.

It is a grim prognosis but, because at thirty-six I am relatively young and because I have no major symptoms, I have a fighting chance of being in that less than one in ten. It makes me uncomfortable to feel that there is nothing I can do to influence my fate.

I am simply not ready to die, not anywhere near it. There are people who talk about the phases of terminal illness, about denial, rage, grief and acceptance, but I do not feel ready to start all that yet. Life is too good, too full of potential, full of people and things I want to see develop, for me to think about giving up on it.

So I went to the holistic treatment centre to see if they had any positive ideas. It was a lovely, relaxing place to spend time and the food was wonderful. I was there for two days, during which time I heard an explanation of how the mind is linked to the body and, in particular, the connection between the mind and the immune system.

The idea behind all of the relaxation, visualisation, healing and nutritional techniques seemed to be that a relaxed, happy and well-nourished person is better able to fight the progress of cancer. It seemed fairly logical, even if some of the techniques did not strike much of a chord with me.

I made some follow-up appointments when I got home and so now, besides chi gong, I am doing daily visualisation exercises and seeing a psychotherapist every week to try to work out how best to minimise stress in my life.

The way I see it is that the worst that can come out of it is that I end up a bit more relaxed and a bit more out of pocket than I would otherwise have been. And if it does help me live a longer and happier life, then it will have been well worth the effort and expense.

Of course I will remain under the care of my main cancer doctor and will take his advice if and when I need more chemotherapy or whatever else. No one at the holistic place was suggesting otherwise. But my real hope remains in the scientists and doctors working on a treatment which has the potential to stop my tumour in its tracks for good.

I have to work carefully and quietly to stay well while they work hard to refine their techniques to the point where they can get a licence for what they do. Relaxing and being happy while all that is going on is not easy but I have to try.

Friday 15 August 2003

I was not in very good shape this time last year. I was having headaches so strong that they made me wake up in the morning and throw up. By the end of the week, I was in hospital and within a day knew that there was a serious problem inside my head.

A few more days and some exploratory brain surgery later, I was told the crushing news that I had a highly malignant brain tumour which would not benefit from surgery. I came home before August was out, paralysed by shock, unable to concentrate and haunted by the fear of death.

It all seems so long ago now. In the meantime I have had aggressive radiotherapy with follow-up chemotherapy and the tumour is apparently at bay. I have grappled to find a way of carrying on.

At first I was so scared that I did not want to know anything but the bare minimum about my condition. I was terrified that someone would tell me that I was bound to die. But it was impossible to bury my head in the sand forever, and the truth came out in dribs and drabs. Once I discovered how poor the statistical chances of surviving three or even five years were, it came as a strange comfort.

I had imagined them to be even worse. The fact is that though they are terrifying, they are not zero, and that is all that matters. If one person in twelve survives, then I will be the one who does. With the help of my wife, my little eighteen-month-old daughter and some professionals, I have slowly learned to live again.

It is not easy to live a happy life in the face of such dreadful uncertainty, but it is possible. Our little girl has gone from a babe in arms to an opinionated, strong-willed person in her own right, sure of what she wants and rapidly developing the ability to express it.

And I have finally made my peace with the idea that I simply do not know what the future holds for me, and that the only thing I can make a good or bad job of is the present.

At the moment I am working full-time, relishing London's long days and summer weather, and looking forward to a day with my family at the seaside tomorrow. I began writing about what happened to me almost as soon as I came out of hospital, at first every week and then, after the first good news about my treatment, every month.

Looking back I can come up with reasons why I was so keen to write this diary, but at the time it was more instinct that made me want to do it – an urge to keep going and to try to make something good come out of something bad.

Now I am going to stop writing.

I hope I managed to accomplish what I set out to do. There have been many kind e-mails from people who have said that what I have written has helped them understand what people close to them are going through.

Whatever the future holds, my cancer diagnosis has not meant the end of my life. What I need to do now is quietly to carry on living, in hope and fear, to be a good husband and father, and to take the greatest of pleasure in all life still has to offer.

12

Me Again

I hoped so much that I would have no cause to write this diary again, if not forever then certainly for a long time after I signed off in August. But that is not the way things turned out.

In August I had been in remission for many months, was fit and well, had been back at work since January and was only occasionally scared about the future. Now I have a serious problem and I need an operation to fix it.

I have been feeling strange for three weeks or so. I have been slightly light-headed, had more trouble than normal seeing my computer screen and had trouble concentrating.

Pretty minor stuff, I thought, and after a few days off work I was beginning to feel better. But my cancer specialist told me to come in for another brain scan anyway and I was stunned by what he said. A watery mess has grown around my tumour and it looks as if a small part of the tumour at least is active and growing once again.

Without an operation the pressure inside my head will just get worse and cause more damage to my brain than I already have from last year. But I am optimistic about what the operation might achieve. If it goes well then I might be back in remission soon, perhaps with the tumour virtually eradicated and firmly under control for a long time to come.

On Tuesday I met the surgeon who will do the operation and he said many confidence-inspiring and encouraging things. The tumour is easily accessible at the back of my head, he said, and not close to any vital structures. I had been labouring under the illusion that my entire brain was a vital structure.

The watery mess around the tumour ought to make it easier to separate from my healthy brain cells. And once all the removal work is done he will pack the space left in my brain with a substance which will release powerful chemotherapy drugs straight on to any remaining bits of tumour. It is a pretty new technique and I am lucky to get access to it.

The operation is on 17 November and if all goes well I will be out of hospital in time for our first wedding anniversary a week later.

I will have a sizable scar to show off, together with titanium clips holding the back of my head together. It will not be pretty but I really hope and believe that it will be good for me.

I have got plenty of living to do yet.

Friday 14 November 2003

I am back in hospital, somewhat earlier than expected.

The operation to try to remove my tumour and relieve the pressure inside my brain is still scheduled for Monday. But I got a nasty headache on Wednesday and the surgeon decided to take me in for observation. My plan, perhaps a little overambitious, had been to go to an old friend's birthday party in Berlin before flying back for the op.

The reason for the headache was a pretty annoying blunder.

Since this last bout of aggravation I have been taking a steroid called dexamethasone. It has some weird side effects but it is very good at controlling swelling and gives me a peaceful head.

But, for most of the last two weeks, I have been taking entirely the wrong drug. My local pharmacist dispensed something with a very similar name.

What he gave me did nothing for my head but would have been great had I had high blood pressure. I understand these things happen more often than people think.

After all that, I am very clearly in the calm before the storm. From my bed I can see the London Eye rotating and the planes coming in to land at Heathrow. A flock of birds has just flown past at the same level as my eighth-floor window.

I have just washed down the first set of tablets, the right ones this time, with a cup of tea.

Before I came in to hospital, I had a few busy days.

I have consistently put off making a will and writing letters to my family. So this week I did those things and I feel better for it.

I have great confidence in the operation I am about to have, but given that any operation carries a small risk, it seemed stupid to be totally unprepared.

I wrote to each of my closest family and I made a film for my daughter. It is a very difficult and painful business to try to compress everything you would like to say to your growing daughter in the future into less than ten minutes of film. I hope that she never sees it.

I will write again after the operation.

Thursday 20 November 2003

I have had my second brain operation, a much more substantial procedure than last time. From what I can tell, it seems to have been a success. Much, if not all, of the bad stuff is gone now.

But I am weak, shocked and drained by the experience. I hope to go home on Friday. I very much want to be home for our wedding anniversary on Sunday. I suspect it will be a fairly sedate affair.

I really have to calm down now, relax and start to feel better. But calm is not easy to come by when you cannot help wondering what the future will bring. I have not really got used to the fact that I have had a relapse. The kind of tumour I have does tend to relapse, so it was not unusual, though obviously I was hoping for much longer before it did.

It is hard not to bargain with time. I say to myself, if I make it to mid-January then our little girl will be two. It does not help but I cannot seem to stop it entirely. I need to go slowly and surely now, rest and exercise.

Monday 24 November 2003

I am out of the hospital and happy as Larry. I am really sorry for the maudlin tone of my last contribution. For two days after the operation I was really shaky, upset and frightened, and then, suddenly the whole thing lifted.

I have had to face facts. I am not going to live forever and there is no cure for what I have.

But that does not matter right now. What matters is that my relapse has been dealt with successfully. My tumour has been removed and an insurance policy has been taken out in the form of chemotherapy applied directly to the brain.

It is cutting-edge stuff, not long available in Britain. I feel great and the inside of my head is in a better state than it has been for the last two years. I am surprised and delighted with the lack of trauma from the operation. There was real fear in my mind before the operation.

But the worst pain has been having the hairs pulled off my arms when they ripped the tape off that held all the anaesthesia lines on. I need nothing more than paracetamol to deal with the post-operative pain.

It has been a much easier ride than I expected and the care in the hospital was first-rate. Now what I need to do is build my strength up and build my confidence moving around. My eyesight has worsened markedly as a result of the relapse and I need to get used to that and compensate for it. I want to look for some training if such a thing exists.

I need to get back on a healthy diet (the Chinese takeaway factor has crept back in) and get back to doing all the exercise and meditation I did before this bout of drama came along.

My good mood is enhanced by the fact that we have just celebrated our first wedding anniversary. We ate cake in a café where we often went before our daughter was born and had an early night. Life is really good and I am glad that I have realised my blessings once again.

From: Tabitha, UK

I was so sorry to hear your latest news – but hang in there. I know you'll come through this with the same fighting spirit you've shown so far. Remember that titanium is very fashionable these days!

From: Di, England

Good luck, Ivan. Following breast cancer, I am having an op to reconstruct. Having followed your journey so far I know exactly what you're going through. I'm sending cyber hugs and prayers to you and your family – think of it this way, we'll both be chucking up from anaesthetic together!

From: Jason Bright, UK

No doubt you've had thousands of messages of support. I just wanted to add mine. As the father of an eighteen-month-old little girl, I can only imagine the stress, pain and anxiety you are going through. I hope the op is successful and enables you to get back to your family as quickly as possible.

From: Pete Kaiser, UK

I hope that if and when I ever have to face something of such magnitude in my life that I have as much strength of mind and as optimistic and positive an outlook as you do. Don't apologise for sounding maudlin – all along you've told it as it is, downs as well as ups. Keep fighting, keep smiling and keep enjoying your family and life.

From: Zoe, Japan

I'm glad that you are out of hospital and feeling better. Don't feel you have to apologise for feeling down or what you wrote – it's natural and human to have good and bad moments/days. Just try to keep focusing on the positive and enjoy what you are doing now – which it sounds like you are already doing. Happy anniversary!

13

Fear of Flying

Friday 5 December 2003

Twelve days out of hospital now and my high spirits persist. I feel really well and everyone keeps telling me how surprised they are that it has been such a quick recovery from the operation.

I was a bit nervous about seeing the surgeon for a follow-up appointment on Tuesday, worried that he might have some lab results with nasty surprises. But there was nothing to worry about. He told me to go and enjoy my Christmas and come back for a brain scan at the end of January to see how everything has settled down.

I am having a whale of a time at the moment, quite frankly. Something interesting happens every day and I meet someone for lunch or tea every day. My wife and my mother have been reminding me that I have had a serious operation and should be taking it easy, but I cannot do it. Time is precious and I cannot sit at home reading a book and quietly sipping tea.

A time may come soon where shopping in town by myself and dropping in on friends at work is no longer possible.

If I am honest, I know that that time could come next year. So I am afraid rest is having to take a back seat.

This weekend I am finishing the steroids I was taking to control the tumour. That might calm me down a bit.

Of course I have started planning some trips, first up to Leeds to see my parents with my daughter, then to Wales with some old friends for three nights before Christmas. We plan spending Christmas itself at home. Our little girl will appreciate it this year, I think, now that she is nearly two. Last year we did not have a tree or anything but I think this year it is a must. Then we are planning to go to Bavaria to spend New Year with two sets of German friends and, with luck, see some snow.

I have been prompted by an e-mail from someone who read this diary recently to think again about the decision I originally took last year not to reveal the details of my diagnosis. I kept it to myself because I was so frightened when I read about what had happened to other people that I thought that I did not want to be the cause of such pain to anyone else.

Now I think that I was wrong and that it would help people affected by tumours to know what I have if they want to judge the severity of what I have. So here it is: I have a grade 4 glioma, otherwise known as glioblastoma multiforme, in my left occipital region (visual cortex).

It was drained of fluid during a burrhole biopsy in August 2002, irradiated with 60 Gray and then I had four cycles of temozolomide, all of which left me in remission until October 2003, when I was made aware that I needed surgical removal of the tumour and a newly-grown fluid cyst.

I had a craniotomy to achieve that, during which the surgeon inserted Gliadel wafers, a mechanism for delivering powerful chemotherapy directly to the brain tissue.

It really is quite remarkable what can be done even for someone with the highest grade of tumour, like me. Fifteen months after diagnosis I am walking around perfectly normally with a smile on my face and the firm conviction that there is plenty of mileage in me yet.

Thursday 11 December 2003

Over the weekend I stopped taking steroids and it really feels good. The drug I was taking – dexamethasone – does a great job of controlling the kind of swelling I had inside my head before last month's operation. But the side effects are pretty powerful too.

My main problem was feeling hectic and impatient all the time and not being able to sleep more than about four or five hours a night. Coming off steroids like dexamethasone has to be done gradually and I seem to have managed it.

Going to bed before midnight and being woken by my daughter just before eight instead of waking by myself at six after dropping off at two is bliss. No longer am I keeping Margaret Thatcher hours, rattling away on the computer in the middle of the night and e-mailing my brother in Hong Kong.

And along with proper sleep comes an all-round feeling of greater normality. Normality, the feeling of being at home and knowing what to do next and what is likely to happen next, is a precious thing.

I have come over all practical and I am trying to sort out my finances, the aim being to keep as much money away from the taxman as possible when I finally bow out. I went to see a financial adviser who opened my eyes as to how little I know about looking after money and what a catastrophic mess I would make of it if left to my own devices. What emerges clearly is that I am good at spending it, rather than saving it, something my wife has long known but I have been loath to admit.

My colleagues at work sent me a very generous present while I was in hospital and I have spent it on buying an extra hard drive for my Mac so that I can edit the video we shot of our little girl when she was first born. It is great fun cutting it all together and captioning it, though I am painfully aware of how terrible I am at shooting video.

Looking back on the last two years reminds me how slow time has become for me. My daughter is not yet two but yet I can barely recall what life felt like without her and even things which happened a year ago feel as if they happened four or five years ago. People say to me, 'Is it really a year?' when they find out I have been married a year but to me it feels far longer ago than that.

It is a function of stress and the amount of drama and crisis we have experienced, I am sure. And it is a great comfort. Knowing that weeks can feel like months and that seasons can feel like years is something to savour when time is not something you can rely on.

Monday 22 December 2003

I have been spending my time doing one of my favourite things. I have been unwrapping and setting up a new computer. Fortunately for our family budget, it is not mine.

It is a friend's fortieth birthday present and he asked me to help with it. I was only too happy. I love installing software on a brand new machine and this one is so fast it's astonishing.

Much of the rest of the time I have been reading a book another friend gave me. It is the autobiography of a Second World War Spitfire pilot. Not my usual reading, but my friend is another person who has been through the cancer mill and he was very keen on it so I thought it was worth a try.

The book is *First Light* by Geoffrey Wellum. It is a great tale but I think what we both got out of reading it, besides it being a good yarn, was being able to look at life through the eyes of someone who did not expect to live very long.

The author manages to get the fear across but also the joy and peace he experiences in the air. I would not want to make too many comparisons to what I am going through, but some of what he had to say struck a chord.

Fear is something which I can never escape from but it does not have to dominate my life, even though if I think about the future, it is frankly terrifying. I have learned to deal with fear and to escape it for most of the time. What I am frightened of is the unknown future. So all I have to do is stay busy enough for there to be too much on my mind to think of the future.

It really works.

I have noticed that I never feel scared when I am doing something like changing my daughter's nappy or cooking the dinner. Things like chi gong and meditation have the same effect. They take me out of myself and give me something to focus on.

I never have trouble filling my time, even though I am not at the office at the moment. I get through books at a rate of knots. I used to worry that all this activity was a form of living a lie and ignoring my condition, but it is not. It is just about having a good time now and to hell with worrying about what comes next.

Thursday 25 December 2003

It has been an uncomfortable week, but I am glad it is Christmas nevertheless.

I wrote a couple of weeks ago about coming off the steroid drugs I was taking to control the swelling in my head left over from the operation five weeks ago. Well, it looks like I came off them too early. I have had a week of scary headaches and a week of worrying what they could be.

Each day I have been waking up with pressure in the left-hand side of my head, across my scar, and a peculiar mark across my left field of vision. It is always difficult to know what to do for the best when something like this happens. The sensible thing, of course, is to phone my doctor and ask for advice. But given the magnitude of what he might tell me, a big part of me wants to wait and see what happens and hope it goes away. And oddly, my little troubles have a habit of falling on a bank-holiday.

I hate waiting for brain scans and appointments for results so it always takes me a few days to summon up the courage to call. This time I phoned him after a week of putting up with the discomfort and the news has been relatively good. I do not have to have a scan just yet, just back on steroids for a little longer and hope that everything calms down soon.

It would have been best if the swelling had disappeared quickly after the operation but even if it takes a bit longer and I have to put up with the hyperactive side effects of the drugs then it is a minor thing in the scheme of things. I should still make my trips to Germany and Scotland in the New Year.

The only worry for today now is what has happened to the Beagle 2 lander on Mars. I have been fascinated by what my colleagues have written about the mission. The little craft has made it over so many obstacles that I find it hard to believe that it may have fallen at the final hurdle.

I will definitely be staying up to see if the second signal comes in on Christmas night and I will have everything crossed that the lander really has made it down safely to the Martian surface.

Reflection — Joe Lister

My sister Jessica was a high-achieving 25-year-old doctor when she noticed something wrong. Before long, she self-diagnosed that she had multiple sclerosis, but it wasn't – a scan showed she actually had a brain tumour the size of an egg. Her doctors didn't know the best way forward for her treatment, and because she herself knew what the result might be, it was eight months before she had surgery. Because her tumour was so large, after the operation she lost a lot of feeling on her left-hand side, and as a person she kind of lost her edge.

She had always been the big sister to me and my brother, and so for us there was suddenly a lot of growing up to do. I particularly felt the need to look after my parents, because they were putting all their energy into looking after Jessica. And even though she tried to be strong for us all, the way she had always been, I have since found out some of what was really going through her mind in those months.

After she died I read some of her diaries from the time. Although outwardly she was trying to lead her life as normally as possible, inside she really was scared. She would have panic attacks, and would wonder what the hell was going on. Some days she was so scared she didn't know how she was going to get up in the morning.

This came as a real shock. I had never heard my sister say she was frightened. You know your siblings through and through, and yet when something like this happens you realise you only know a slice of them – you probably don't know the person they are with their friends or their boyfriend or girlfriend. You certainly don't know their darkest fears.

I wish I had talked to her more about her feelings, but the thing you are told again and again is that you shouldn't treat someone who is dealing with a tumour any differently from the way you would normally treat them. So you tend not to bring up their fears – in any case, you want to be strong for them, certainly not bring them down. But looking back I just wish I had spent more time talking. Like lots of people in this situation, I just thought we would have more time. I didn't think she would die so soon.

That's one of the reasons I wrote to Ivan in March 2003. I told him about finding Jessica's diaries and how amazing it had been to discover that she had been as human and scared as the people who loved her. British people, like my family, often don't find it easy to talk openly, so I felt that in some way reading Ivan's diary had helped me have an insight into some of what Jessica might have been feeling.

14

Another New Beginning

Thursday 15 January 2004

On Thursday my little girl turns two. A large strawberry gateau is in preparation as I write. And given her current obsession with fire engines, I have no doubt what she will be unwrapping in the morning.

When I was diagnosed, she was just six months old. She has been a focus for my fears for this past year-and-a-half, and that has not been easy. But with all her charm, curiosity, joy and laughter, she has made me enormously happy and repeatedly grateful that she is part of our lives.

We have spent the New Year in Bavaria, where she got to grips with proper snow and sledging. Bavaria in the snow looked like a picture postcard and the food there was irresistible.

The big news, though, is that it seems our daughter has a sister on the way. My wife is three months' pregnant and the monographer who did the 12-week scan was fairly sure that the baby is a girl. I am of course utterly delighted.

The news was hard to digest though when it first arrived,

coming as it did at the same time that I realised I was relapsing and needing the operation I had in November.

Deciding whether to try to have another child was not easy. I was very worried about whether it was right to bring a child into the world in the knowledge that if the statistics came true for me, it would never remember its father. And I was worried about how my wife would cope if I died before or soon after the birth.

But at the same time I had a strong gut feeling that I wanted to fight death with life. And as a friend has said since, my parents' generation was born in the middle of a world war. My wife and I both thought that our children would be happier if there were more than one of them.

I hope most of all that I will be able to spend as much time as possible with my children, but if things do not go as well as I hope, then I hope that they will understand why we decided what we did.

The chemotherapy I had and the mutations it may have caused to my sperm meant that we had to use sperm I had frozen before I was treated. Taking such a deliberate and mechanical approach to conception was a far cry from the joyful coincidence we experienced the first time. But we were lucky and it worked quickly, far more quickly than we expected. I could not help being rather proud that my sperm had survived a year in liquid nitrogen.

Once again, we have much to be grateful for, and plenty to worry about. It is going to be an interesting year.

Friday 6 February 2004

I have had a real setback.

I had a brain scan on Monday and it showed that my tumour had regrown a big chunk, despite the operation I had only two-and-a-half months ago to remove it. It is a big blow. We hoped that the operation and the drugs that went in with it would have kept me stable for a lot longer.

Our thoughts, of course, are on our growing baby. There are five-and-a-half months to go before the birth of my second child, but what does that mean when my tumour is growing at such a rate?

The operation to remove chunks of the cancer can be repeated but, as the surgeon made clear to me, each time is riskier and less effective than the last. We think that it is worth a try, though, so later this month I will have the operation again, followed by some traditional chemotherapy which worked well for someone else in a similar case. The hope is that the surgery will buy time and the chemotherapy will bring on a return to remission.

At the moment I am having trouble coming to terms with it all. The speed of events is bewildering and I had not bargained on dealing with all this right now. I had learned to deal with the fear that comes with the uncertainty of my illness but suddenly it is back, intrusively.

There are two weekends and a week before the operation. I am going to try to relax and take a trip with my wife and my little girl, and get on with the thing that makes sense: having a good time while it lasts.

Friday 13 February 2004

I am very happy to be writing this in Berlin. We decided to do something good before my next operation, which is on Tuesday. We arrived in falling snow on Tuesday but the weather has now cleared and is cold and crisp. A new aquarium has opened in the centre of town and it was a great hit with our daughter when we took her there on Wednesday. I first came to Berlin as a student fifteen years ago and spent nearly two years here.

I learned most of my German here, lived and worked in the east and crossed the Berlin Wall the night it fell. I got my first

BBC job as a result, and I am a happy man when I am back here. The last couple of times we have tried to come we have had to cancel, so I am especially pleased to have made it.

We fly back on Saturday to enjoy a couple more days' recreation before the op. Life now is going to be about snatching as much as we can and hoping for the best. The operation is about buying time.

The chemotherapy that follows may buy more time, possibly quite a lot if it does work at all. But we are being realistic.

By the time our new baby comes, in July if all goes well, I may be very unwell or worse. Some powerful medication is keeping me well at the moment and it will not keep going forever. I am not sad about what is happening, which surprises me at times. I am not angry either.

It is not that I am not an angry person. I am frequently angry, but I think I need someone to get angry with and there is no one to blame for my cancer, only lots of people who help me with it. Whenever we get bad news, I am shocked for a while but after a few days we seem to readjust to the new situation and carry on. I am determined that we will make as much as we can out of what we have left.

No doctor expects me to recover from this cancer and I think that I can accept that now without a feeling that I am giving up. Accepting the dangers does not mean giving up.

A miracle may happen and the tumour may suddenly stop growing. These things happen to some people but the probability is minuscule. The best comfort I have of course is that I am with the people I love, am having a good time and am walking around on my own two feet. I have no idea how long that will go on, but that is itself a comfort and every day is a pleasure.

And I think I will see the new baby. I have a good feeling.

Judging by how I felt immediately after my last operation, it will be difficult for me to write to say how it went. I was pretty confused and upset for a short while last time. I will write as soon as I feel myself again, or ask someone to write a couple of lines for me.

From: Rachel Garner, Brighton

I am sorry to hear about the latest news but know that the strength of character which has already shone through will give you the courage to go on. I am currently in remission from cancer of the lymph glands and have a two-and-a-half-year-old son. I know where your deepest fears lie and would share with you one line from a wonderful Macmillan counsellor. I was worried that I may not be able to be Jacob's mummy in the future and she said: 'You will always be his mummy.' These words comforted me enormously at a time of great uncertainty - I hope they may do the same for you.

From: Sheila, England

Many congratulations on the blessings of a new baby on the way. I hope your children inherit your spirit, you sound as if you are well named. Nobody would choose to go through what you have to but I hope the love and good wishes you receive from people who feel they know you bring you strength.

From: Lynda Hurst, Canada

You've made a wise choice in having a
second child. And I trust you will be
there for a long while yet to enjoy her
as much as your first daughter. All good
wishes to you and your wife.

From: Dumisani Phakathi, Soweto, South Africa

Akulahlwa mbeleko ngakufelwa - this is a
famous Zulu saying which is meant to
restore hope during difficult times.

From: Ann Smith, UK

I have never had to face what you have
had to face but maybe you can take some
encouragement from a motto I adopted some
time ago (courtesy of Charles Schulz).
'Live for today, plan for tomorrow, party
tonight' - it is all any of us can do
really to make the most of the gift of
life.

From: Jaq McDiarmid, Scotland

My husband introduced me to your story
when my dad was in the middle of his own
fight with cancer. He had your
determination but I just wish he'd had
your openness to discuss his feelings and
emotions. Keep your loved ones involved
as you are doing and that way they know
they're fighting this huge battle with
you.

From: Ben, Norway

My wife is pregnant with our first child
at the moment, while her mother has
cancer and this contrast between new life
and uncertain future is amazing to
experience, amazing to think about. You
can be assured that your second child
will be proud to be your daughter even if
she never meets you – and I sincerely
wish that she does – I'll pray that she
does.

15

An Extra Shot

I am back from the surgery and, though still in hospital, feeling better than I thought possible. We had been ready for some difficult days. Three months ago when I had my second operation I was pretty confused and upset for a couple of days before I managed to bounce back.

This time it is quite different. I am happy, comfortable and enjoying my food and I have been back for less than forty-eight hours as I write. I really am pleased.

I'm very grateful to the people looking after me, the medical team and especially to everyone who has been wishing me well. All that goodwill makes a big difference. I have a few days now to spend in hospital recovering and the surgeon says I should be able to go home on Sunday. It is all good news so far.

I am particularly pleased at managing to get out with my wife to the cinema and for dinner before everything kicked off. My parents are looking after our little girl for a few days so we managed to see *Lost in Translation* and then go to a restaurant we have not been to for a long time – a real pleasure.

And then in the morning a very enjoyable double strength latte before I had to go nil by mouth. I am looking forward to being out and about again.

Thursday 26 February 2004

I am out of hospital now and back home, feeling very chipper after what I have to keep reminding myself is my third round of brain surgery. I got home on Saturday lunchtime and have been making a concerted effort to relax and not go rushing around in the general exhilaration at feeling so well.

The kind of operation I have just had is not without its risks and up until three hours beforehand I successfully put them out of my mind as something that I could not influence. Then I panicked, and then I stopped.

Thankfully everything went well and I was babbling away on the anaesthetic asking for phone calls to my wife and parents in no time. Now I am on a real high, delighted to be alive, unscathed and with a bit more time in the bag.

I am still on quite a high dose of steroids after the op, so I am up with the larks. The only problem is that these larks spend a lot of time on early morning Internet shopping, which is starting to take its toll on the family budget.

The next medical thing is some chemotherapy to try to arrest the tumour and buy even more time. I will find out on Thursday when this is to be. In the meantime we have a scan of our growing baby to look forward to and I am also very excited about the impending arrival of my brother from China.

Chemotherapy permitting we have some plans which I hope will keep us both entertained and give my wife a brief break from looking after me, our daughter, her job and her pregnancy all at once.

It has never been easy since that awful day a year-and-a-half ago but somehow I feel I'm coping better now.

In terms of my prognosis, things are more precarious than ever, but there are good reasons for hope still and I have finally learned not to be intimidated by time. I know what I want to do and I am doing it, without fear and doubt, and that makes me feel strong.

Quite frankly, 99 per cent of the time I am having a ball. Long may I be able to keep writing that.

Wednesday 10 March 2004

A lot is happening. I have started chemotherapy much earlier than I expected. Only three weeks have gone by since the operation to remove as much as possible of the tumour growing in the back of my head and already I am well over ten days into the new chemotherapy.

I feel fine. I took five tablets at home over two days and I did not feel sick at all. I have not started feeling tired either, though that is likely to begin soon and last seven to ten days if it comes at all.

I am pleased that I have got started on the treatment so soon but I was shocked, too. I suppose that there is simply no reason to hang about but it did make me think that the doctor was so keen to get started because my tumour is so aggressive.

Anyway, in the meantime I am enjoying life with my brother – he's staying for two weeks, first driving me round England and then keeping me company back in London. We began with the sad task of putting one of our grandmothers to rest at the age of ninety-one. She was very ill and died a couple of days before my operation.

The funeral was sad, but I think we did everything she would have wanted and it was something I will not forget. And our other ninety-one-year-old grandmother is well and was delighted by a rare visit from both her grandchildren at the same time.

After time with our parents in Yorkshire, we went off to a

wonderful hotel near York where we were spoiled with great food and a massage each.

Then on to friends in Sowerby Bridge, a dash south to a christening in Southampton, and an impromptu rendezvous with a friend of my brother's, who is about to spend a year travelling the world with her husband.

Finally lunch at Windsor because it is on the way and I have never been before and then back to Heathrow Airport to collect my wife and daughter, who have been home to Germany.

I am at home now so that the whole of my family can meet up at our place and then on Thursday I am to have a brain scan. The scan itself is not frightening at all, especially having had so many now, but I am never fond of the injection that comes halfway through.

A contrast agent gets put in towards the end to highlight the tumour on the scan and often they cannot get the dye to go in properly. It really hurts when that happens and they have to start again. And you cannot see the person sticking the needle in because you are inside the machine. This week's scan was described as a baseline scan, so it is not expected to show any changes, but rather to tell us what the inside of my head looks like after the operation.

But for one reason or another, quite a bit of time will have passed between the operation and the scan and so it may show something. In any case it will be quite a few days before I am told anything.

Our baby continues to wriggle and grow and the last scan was very good but we had an enormous shock when we asked if we could be told the sex. We had been told at twelve weeks that she was most probably a girl and we had begun to contemplate Rosalind as a name, after the DNA pioneer Rosalind Franklin. But now she has revealed herself very definitely as a boy.

I am very happy. With all this treatment underway, too, I feel more optimistic about my chances of spending time with him. Now we are back to the question of names.

From: Camilla, England

As one of the countless 'out there' in
Internet-land, I anxiously reach for your
diary the minute I see it mentioned on-
screen. Keep going, keep being strong and
cheerful, we need your warmth and wisdom
to inject a little humility into our
complacent lives. And I'm sure your
family need you even more. They are lucky
to know you, and we are lucky to have
you share your experiences with us.

From: Alison, Scotland

Ivan, what wonderful news about your son.
Having lost my father to cancer four
years ago I know that your brave decision
to have another child was absolutely the
right one. I don't know how I would have
coped without my brother to support me.
Whatever happens in your (hopefully long
and healthy) future I'm sure your
daughter will be glad to have a brother.
As for names I think Franklin Noble
definitely has a certain ring to it.

From: Mike Reed, England

Thank you for sharing your bravery. If
your son has half your spirit he will
make an impact on the world. Perhaps you
should call him Ivan; he will thank you
for it when he reads your diary. I wish
you a full recovery.

From: Mike Harlow, UK

Thanks for so publicly demonstrating that everyday life can be so savoured. I'm always too busy complaining about speed bumps and time flying and taxes and English cricket and work and bills and bad TV and the youth of today to have time to appreciate life.

From: Trevor Martin, USA/UK

I am inspired by your thoughts and feelings. I was diagnosed with full blown AIDS three years ago and it has taken me the full three years to get over the shock and to wrestle down those feelings of fear, no doubt similar to those feelings you've mentioned. Although we live in more optimistic times now with regard to AIDS and HIV, it is still a chastening experience to be confronted with one's own vulnerability and to be forced to face some of life's most challenging questions.

From: Clare, Australia

Keep strong with your 'realistic optimism'. Life is uncertain, eat dessert first!

Reflection – Jeanie Veris

I first wrote to Ivan in January 2003, a month before my husband Peter died from the same kind of tumour, a GBM. I wrote then that his wife would find many unknown strengths, but like me she wouldn't mind one bit, as love comes above everything.

Peter's situation was pretty different, not least because his tumour was in his frontal lobe which meant his personality changed as his cancer worsened. He became very unpredictable – for instance, when he wanted things he wanted them there and then. Fortunately for what was to come, he also developed a very childlike, happy-go-lucky outlook.

But one of the biggest differences was that Peter never knew the seriousness of his cancer. In retrospect perhaps we should have realised, but after his first operation, we thought it had been removed; when he then had radiotherapy, we were told it was just in case there were any microbes left. A few months later, though, I found out the name of the type of tumour. I looked it up online, and yes, like Ivan, I got the fright of my life. I just didn't have the courage to tell Peter what I had found out. I had to put on a big act which lasted two years.

I tried to talk to the doctors about it, but they couldn't speak to me unless Peter was present. So every time we went for an appointment, I would be thinking: 'Perhaps they'll tell him today?' But they never did. And as Peter was in denial about it anyway, he just wasn't interested in asking questions.

It became a very lonely experience, being the only person who knew. I think in a lot of cases, the friends and family of someone with a tumour just don't know how to give the right support. Only a few of his friends stayed with us, but then I could hardly go round telling them that his cancer was terminal when he didn't even know himself, so they didn't know how bleak things were looking. The normality of life which everyone else took for granted had been taken away from us.

Eleven months before he died, he was very ill and we thought he was about to leave us. He and I had been living together for years, but a Macmillan nurse suggested to Peter that we could get married in the hospice, which we did. It was such a beautiful time, and has given me the most wonderful memories. Peter attended hospice day care weekly for a year, which he thoroughly enjoyed. People think hospices are where you go to die, but anyone who's ever visited one will know what amazing places they are – there's no sense of fear there, just a fantastic peace.

Since he died, I have become chairperson of our local brain tumour support group, and I've spent a lot of time thinking and talking about brain tumours. It seems to me that these kinds of tumours are more common than you might think, and that there are pockets around the country where they seem to occur more frequently. Treatment is ineffective in most cases and research is underfunded for this type of tumour. I've now gone to university, aged forty-one, to do a degree in social work and mental health nursing – ultimately I want to work alongside the Macmillan nurses, and add a social work element to the excellent work they do.

But the biggest lesson for me in all this, just as I suspect it might be for Ivan, is that it can happen to anyone. Thirty-three-year-old Peter, a chef-turned-taxi-driver, woke up one day and it was there. It's as simple as that.

16

Fighting for Time

Things are getting harder.

My brain scan this week was very encouraging in the short term. It showed that although my tumour is still there and active, there is space at the moment for it to grow.

I breathed a sigh of relief as I heard because I knew it meant that I could relax for a couple of weeks. My next appointment is just before Easter as I start another cycle of chemotherapy. It would be wonderful if the chemo could halt the tumour for a while, a significant while even.

And even if it does not, I could have yet another operation to reduce the size of the tumour. That would be a worry but at least finally a chance to roll out my 'I need another craniotomy like I need a hole in the head' joke.

But I have now faced up to the fact that I am fighting for time. Miracles do happen, but by definition extremely rarely, and without one this tumour is going to kill me sooner or later.

Everything is uncertain now and I am as positive and keen to fight on as ever, but I would be deceiving everyone if I did not face up to the truth. My immediate battle is to see the birth of my son, due in July. The tumour is such an aggressive one that getting to July in any fit state to participate is a big fight. I am ready for it but I also have had to start preparing myself for what will happen if I lose.

I put off thinking about dying for as long as I could and I really did not allow it into my thinking until my tumour removal operation in November 2003. While I was still in hospital, my favourite nurse asked me something along the lines of whether I was worried about anything. He was meaning whether I was comfortable and had any pain but I flippantly answered, 'Dying of cancer'.

He took the question seriously and said some very sensitive and helpful things but it was still a shock and made me think for the first time that it was something for which I had to prepare. Four months later the process is much further on.

I can talk about my death practically and rationally. If at times I panic about it, the panic passes and I know how to deal with it and get back on track. I can cry about it and I can laugh about it and accepting its inevitability has made me feel stronger, less afraid and more in control.

The time ahead is an entirely uncertain one, but most of the time I am happy and full of ideas of what we can do with our time. Soon I will be leaving for another week in the Scottish highlands with my wife, daughter and some friends. As long as we can, we will be fitting the treats in between the medical appointments and, I hope, creating memories that will last long after I have gone.

And for as long as I can I will still be writing my diary. It has always been part of fighting the tumour. I started it to make something positive out of a calamity and for me it has preserved a link to a job I was proud of doing. All the fantastic e-mails have been a great boost and they continue to be. I am lucky to be able to have such a project.

One final thing about terminal illness: sometimes when people mention advanced cancer they use that term. It is not one I accept for myself yet. I will accept it only when my doctors, friends and family have run out of ideas and I cannot fight any more. There is so much we have left to do in whatever time we manage to steal from this thing.

So I am going downstairs to make a coffee and to continue to steal shamelessly for as long as I can.

Monday 29 March 2004

I am writing at dawn, watching the light grow over water and snow-capped hills in a beautiful and remote part of the western highlands of Scotland. I am looking forward to another day here entertaining our two-year-old, who is utterly unfazed by the sudden move from London's stress and bustle to a place where we are observed by stags and highland cattle.

And of course, if I am honest, what is really going on is that she is entertaining us. Accompanied by a friend a few months older, the stream of hilarity and the sheer level of energy is impressive. Fortunately there are plenty of us here to soak it up.

And being here has begun to soak up the stress and tension of what I have to deal with in a way that must be as good for me as all the other treatment. The people involved in organising this trip, transporting me here, hosting my stay and keeping me company know who they are and I am taking this liberty to add a public thank you to the private ones.

What I have begun to notice is that as things become more uncertain and life becomes more and more intense, my perception of things is changing.

I feel as if I have lost the middle range of my opinion of things. I think everything is either fantastic or terrible. There is rarely an in-between. The trip here is genuinely magical. But something like a trip to see an undemanding and slushy film will have me delighted and trying to discuss the quality of the film with my wife before I realise that she and probably everyone else in the cinema has a less rapturous view of Jennifer Aniston's efforts.

I saw some colleagues from work before I left for Scotland and, again, enjoyed myself hugely. But it struck me after I left how odd it must be for them to have this steroid-fuelled monster turn up talking nineteen to the dozen, crashing in to their working lives to tell them probably more than they needed to know about the madnesses of my world. I had great fun, though, and am sorry only for the people I wanted to see and missed.

With the enthusiasms come the rages.

The doorbell rings and it is someone trying to sell something, but refusing to acknowledge the fact, posing instead as a new neighbour who coincidentally has a new business starting up. At the time I am with a nurse working to collect data from me for a huge study to investigate the possible causes of my tumour. Never a patient person, I have to slam the door on the intruder before the F-word escapes my lips.

I have no time for such nonsense.

But my special rage is saved for my bank. Until a while ago, they used to ring me up to try to sell me things which a simple check of my account would have told them were entirely inappropriate. They did it in a really irritating way, cold-calling and refusing to discuss anything, saying only which bank they were and asking for security details before they would go further.

Quite apart from the fact that it should have been them identifying themselves, not the customer, it gives the impression that the call is important. If you are daft enough to go along with it, as I have been too many times, it is on to the real time-wasting.

After several attempts I was designated something I think they call 'telephone contact unresponsive' and they finally stopped the nonsense.

Until now.

They are back and I am afraid I flew into an incandescent rage this time. I slammed the phone down at the end and then spent ages kicking myself for not saying something more intelligent. Then I went on to compose mental letters to the complaints department until I calmed down far enough to think, 'What a waste of time!' Quite.

Sunday 18 April 2004

I have been doing some odd things. Physically, I feel really good, apart from a stinker of a cold recently acquired from my daughter. But mentally I have been under a lot of stress.

What I have been up to is not that weird in itself – I filled the car up with petrol, which is a bad idea if you own a diesel and it is Easter. An expensively bad idea.

And everyone is at pains to say how they have done it too and how normal it is. But when you are racking up incidents like that on an almost daily basis, you begin to wonder what has happened to your powers of concentration. Facing up to what will happen sooner or later has been much, much tougher than I realised it would be.

It is one thing to write it in a diary, and another to feel the reality of it run through you and the sheer terror short-circuit your brain. I think that I am slowly coming out the other side of this latest episode. I really hope so. It does not make for good company.

I had two medical appointments last week – one a follow-up to the operation two months ago and the other a blood test and consultation to verify that I was strong enough to withstand another round of chemotherapy.

It was the first one which I could not handle. I have not had a brain scan recently so there should have been nothing to be scared of. No scan means no news, which by definition means no bad news. But there are always frightening conversations which might develop.

And I managed to work myself into a real lather before I even walked in. So I came up with a plan to take charge of the situation. I decided all I wanted to do was run through the checks which the consultant always does – basic tests like walking in a straight line to demonstrate that my brain is still working normally – and then I would leave my long-suffering wife to handle the rest of the conversation.

Unfortunately, I was so hyped up about the whole thing that I started gabbling, skipped across the room like a child, then sat down for about a minute until my trigger word – speech – was mentioned, whereupon I ran for it and did not come back.

My embarrassed wife and consultant handled the rest of the session and I still have not had the courage to learn what they discussed.

I was very rude and I owe the two of them an apology. But it does illustrate the power of fear and how different patients have different needs. I have no desire whatsoever to hear anything about what is happening to me or might happen to me unless I need to make an immediate decision about it; for instance, when I had to decide whether or not to have the last operation.

But doctors obviously have a much better idea of what lies ahead, even though they do not control the timing. I know that my tumour is very close to the bit of brain controlling my speech and I know that the reason my consultant mentions my speech every time we meet is that he is concerned that any worsening of my condition will affect it. He is pleased every time he sees me with normal speech because to him it shows I am doing well.

But I have had normal speech for thirty-six years or so and I do not think about it being otherwise unless someone brings the subject up. Hence my undignified exit. I know that I will not survive this disease for a long time, but I would like to be as normal and as comfortable as possible.

That means screwing every last second of pleasure, love, happiness and often general bad behaviour out of the here and now, and not thinking about terrifying developments which may be a month, three months or half a year away. Now is a rewarding, intense, at times very emotional and at times utterly frightening time.

It is a time of rapid psychological change for me and I really hope I am moving towards peace and calm, away from the manic days of the last fortnight. And I hope I am managing to describe it properly.

From: Lyn Hewitt-Jones, Bournemouth, Dorset

I admire your strength and courage in the face of what must seem like overwhelming trials - please do not lose heart, even though the next few weeks will be hard. Just think of July, and a small, shouting baby and all you have to look forward to with your family. God bless.

From: Eliza, USA

Your latest entry has really struck to the core and I wanted to send you a quote that I received today which I feel echoes what I hear you say: 'Life may not be the party we asked for, but as long as we're here, we might as well dance.' Keep on dancing, friend.

From: Stuart, expat in Australia

Your open and candid thoughts about the
cancer you've been inflicted with have
been an inspiration to us all. As a
nurse, I just wanted to say that whatever
happens in the future, your diary should
be used by nursing students around the
world to understand there is a person
behind the patient. You also show that we
are all special, everyone has loves,
lives and people who care about us. If we
all were able to look at our neighbours
in those terms I think conflict would be
very hard to justify.

From: Rob Jacks, England

My best friend passed away at the age of
thirty-two, just before he was due to get
married. He was a fantastic person who I
miss everyday. Your diaries help me
remember the fantastic times my friend
had during his illness. The fact that you
are able to rationally cope and still
spend quality time with those that you
love is fantastic - those memories do go
on forever.

From: George, UK

I wouldn't be too hard on yourself, Ivan.
I spent most of yesterday raging at my
television because for unknown reasons it
was unable to show me the India vs.

Pakistan cricket highlights I had wanted to watch. Eventually, my flatmate called me 'childish' which caused another rage – and plenty of embarrassment when I had to apologise later. More importantly, it's a grey old day here in London and I am very jealous of you in Scotland. Is there anywhere more beautiful in the world?

From: Amanda, UK

Just remember all the special people that are there with you that make you smile. Glad you are having a relaxing time. Keep your chin up.

From: Anon, UK

Even the toughest of people fear the inevitable decline. Never be ashamed of how you are coping with your journey, it's yours. Don't be ashamed of being scared, you are brave to admit your fears. Brave faces hide a mass of emotions. I cannot say don't be scared, because I know I would, and so would many more.

From: Bern Webb, USA

I have discussed your plight with friends here and it is an emotional conversation because we are attached to you now like we're friends, it's as if you have created a community. And as for the

outburst in the doctor's office, I really
wouldn't mind if you had done everything
on a pogo stick. It's OK. Peace to you
from the States.

From: Annabel, Bucks

Ivan, you are handling this just fine.
You don't need to apologise. Really.
Sometimes we cope by 'not coping' and you
seem to be coping marvellously. Who can
blame you for wanting to run away. Ride
that storm, Ivan!

17

Stubbly Grump

Friday 7 May 2004

This is the first time I have written in several weeks.

I have been spending a lot of time asleep. The reason I think is that the side effects of my chemotherapy have finally kicked in in a big way. I am living the quiet life – it is good for me. The first cycle of treatment, which ended well over a month ago, was pretty much unnoticeable until the very end.

But this second cycle has been exactly as predicted, with my hyperactivity giving way to serious lethargy ten days after I took the tablets. Lethargic is the way I have stayed. Before, I was waking between 4 and 6 a.m. with my mind racing, often having finished everything I wanted to write before anyone else in my time zone was awake.

Now I am waking about 7.30, downing the coffee and sweet porridge which I am often delighted to find by my bedside, then falling asleep again before 9 a.m. despite the best efforts of the *Today* programme. I really should turn it up again after 'Thought for the Day'.

Actual dressing rarely happens before lunch and sometimes not at all. The good side of all this has to be that rest must be doing me good. I feel well and everyone else, when they catch me awake, seems to think I look OK. The downside is that the days are just sliding by, with nothing to distinguish one from the next. It really is the case that drama and crisis cause time to slow down, while peace, quiet, rest and lack of calamities make the time go by faster.

Today at least I have moved locations, back to Scotland again, albeit Edinburgh instead of the highlands. I am settling in to a long weekend of relaxation and good company here.

I had half a mind to apologise for this report being so short. But I am not going to. I am really glad that nothing bar a couple of minor headaches have happened to me since I last wrote and that I am living the quiet life. It is good for me. Drama will return in its own good time.

Wednesday 2 June 2004

For a long time I have been trying to put off thinking about the birth of my son.

I have seen him in scans at the hospital and I have felt him moving around. But I have been too scared of what might happen to me before he is born to let myself really look forward to meeting him.

One of the really depressing things about this disease is that it can turn you in upon yourself without you really noticing. Cancer and all that surrounds living with it are such big things that it is easy to lose sight of the lives of other people. Chemotherapy is tiring and sometimes I sit around watching the world go by and waiting for the people who look after me to come and go.

But the lives of the people close to me are part of my future. They are the future that will become the present when I am gone. So it is time now to be a bit braver and play my part.

Medically it looks like I am doing well. I have just started my third six-week cycle of chemotherapy and my blood test results showed I was tolerating it well. And I reached a significant point when I realised it was now more than three months since my last operation.

Three months after my November operation I already needed another. But now three-and-a-half months after my February op I am doing really well, better than expected. I appear to have got through the couple of months where I was really manic. And I am happy that I have managed to reduce my intake of steroids. Steroids are there to suppress the swelling around a tumour and so the fact that I have managed to cut down on them is very good.

Now, then, I am trying to summon up a bit more strength and remember that I have more than one child to think about. We should be able to see our little boy on another ultrasound scan this week. We heard his heartbeat on a monitor last week and it was good and strong. He moves around all the time.

All we can do now is get the house ready for him and make up our minds about his name. It will not be long now – he is due in July.

Friday 18 June 2004

A few days ago I passed another milestone when we celebrated my thirty-seventh birthday. I have always been a great fan of birthdays and this one was especially enjoyable. The three of us and the bump spent it in and around a hotel in Suffolk.

Somehow the celebrations and treats have stretched on for a few days and the whole experience has been lovely. It has lifted my spirits at a time when I have been struggling a bit.

I appear to be responding well to the various things that have been done to keep me going. I should be happy and throwing myself into preparations for the baby, due now in four weeks. And to an extent, I am.

But I have gained a new nickname at home: Stubbly Grump.

'Stubbly' on account of the infrequency of my encounters with a razor blade and 'Grump' for obvious reasons. I have started trying to announce 'My name's Stubbly – Stubbly Grump' like Tom Hanks as Forrest Gump. I can occasionally raise a laugh but more often than not our daughter, by now almost two-and-a-half and ever a stickler for correctness, contests the point, saying: 'No, you're not. You're my daddy.'

Bless her.

Staying positive is a struggle which I seem to have to fight and refight every so often. Dealing with the uncertainty is really hard. I know very well now from experience how quickly I can move from a good phase to needing serious and risky intervention. The answer, of course, is to stay busy, look outwards not inwards and engage with life as it is now instead of worrying about death at some point in the future.

But some mornings that trick is not always an easy one to pull off. While in Suffolk we went to Sutton Hoo to visit the site where seventh-century Saxon treasure was found at the end of the 1930s.

A famous masked helmet found there is in the British Museum, but the site has a newish visitor centre which relates a huge amount of detail about life 1,300 years ago as England was beginning to solidify into a single state.

The burial mounds are still visible after all the centuries and one, destroyed by looters long ago, has been rebuilt to demonstrate how it would have looked in Saxon times. I love the idea that it is possible for someone to have been dead for dozens of generations but still speak to the living through everything that was left behind.

Life then, as for most of the tens of thousands of years of human existence, was hard and frequently short. I imagine reaching thirty-seven then must have been quite an achievement, too.

From: Julie, UK

I first came across your diary when my
husband-to-be was diagnosed with an
ependymoma within his spinal cord last
October. Fortunately his surgery was
successful and the tumour benign and, with
the assistance of on-going OT and physio,
he is now back at work, albeit without
feeling in his lower arms and hands. I
showed Paul your diary today for the first
time as your experience with the bank's
telesales staff were a constant gripe of
his while he was at home recuperating. His
real hate is commuters who would seem to
prefer to push people on to the tracks out
of their way if it would save them a
second on their journey. He too also
becomes emotional at things which, prior
to his diagnosis he would have found
silly. I stared in disbelief as he joined
me shedding tears of joy at the end of
Love Actually and heaven help us if the
underdog wins at *Countdown*! I've enjoyed
reading your diary and think you very
brave to share your experiences. It helped
me through some dark hours and I thank you
for that.

From: Sharon, UK

Keep positive! What keeps me going (I am
recovering from breast cancer) are these
lovely words and of course my wonderful
family and friends.

Yesterday is history
Tomorrow is a mystery
Today is a gift from G-d
And that is why we call it the present

No one knows what the next moment is
going to bring therefore enjoy every
second especially with your wife and
darling daughter. It is all so precious.

From: Matt, UK

Good luck, mate. I've sometimes found it
hard to read your diary – I want to
avoid confronting my own fears of
mortality and serious illness, I
suppose. I think it is a good thing for
you to have done though, brave. Anyway,
I hope you regain some energy and find
some way to make the time pass with more
purpose.

From: Philip Dickinson, UK

Ivan, I have seen you column many times
in the last few months and have ignored
it. Then last week an MRI scan (following
what seemed to be a groin strain)
revealed a growth, possibly a tumour, to
be confirmed soon by biopsy. Suddenly my
focus has come crashing darkly around me
and I am often finding it hard to
participate in simple human interactions.
Actually, there are lots of positives to
bear in mind and there is *no* firm

diagnosis yet, so I will lock down my
fears as best I can for the moment. Your
fight now seems very brave to me.

18

The Shoe Problem

We now have only a day to go until our son is due to be born. All
being well, he should make his move some time in the next two
weeks.

What with a pregnancy, two major brain operations and on-
going treatment of my tumour, we have had plenty of experience
of dealing with the medical profession over the last nine months.
I have written before about my admiration for doctors' skill and
persistence, so I hope I am not too far out of line now deciding to
suggest a few improvements some of them might make.

First of all, the problem of delivering bad news.

No one likes delivering bad news.

I know that I am not the first person to write this, but the shoe
problem still needs dealing with. When delivering bad news, a
doctor really should be looking the patient in the eye, not staring
at his or her own feet.

Bad news is bad news, but I would have felt much less
distressed when I was given my diagnosis had the doctor

concerned spent a little more time explaining what was going to happen to me next and what could be done to help me.

As it was I left hospital in total shock and only slowly began to piece together what my treatment would mean. The doctor who gave me my diagnosis could not wait to get out of the room and hand me over to a nurse.

Looking back now over almost two years, I have dealt with several shocks and I can put things into perspective now. But back at the beginning a little more time and a few more strong, encouraging words would have made that first week so much less painful.

I assume some doctors must feel a sense of failure when they give bad news to a patient. But there has to be another way of looking at it. Whatever the prognosis, there is always some way forward, even if the treatment is palliative rather than curative. And I know from personal experience that when someone did stand in front of me and tell me in a confident tone how my treatment was going to go forward, I felt a whole lot better.

It is easy for doctors to lose sight of what it is like to be a patient. Doctors are part of a system which they understand.

Patients frequently do not understand what is going on. If I go to a new place, I never do. It takes less than a minute to say to a patient: 'I am Dr So-and-so. I am a specialist in dealing with X. I am here to help you with Y problem. Dr Whatsit is the doctor who sent you to me.' But much of the time it never happens.

Doctors dress in a much friendlier way these days, but that does lead to situations where if the doctor does not identify herself as such, no one is the wiser.

And terms like 'SHO' and 'registrar' do not help people who do not habitually hang around hospitals. When someone says 'registrar' to me, I think of Births, Marriages and Deaths.

Patients like to think the doctor knows who they are. Obviously very few doctors can remember all their patients in detail – this is why they have notes. But it really does make a difference to the psychological impact a doctor's care makes on a patient if, before the patient gets through the door, the doctor has scanned through enough of the notes to know what the patient was last seen for and when.

And when patients are nearly always seen by a different doctor each time they come in, there has to be something that can be done to improve continuity. It really is quite disconcerting to go with your partner to an ante-natal check up and to realise that the doctor appears either not to have had time to read the semi-legible notes or not to be able to make sense of what the last person wrote.

The overall impression is of being in a system that expanded by evolution, not design. That is of course inevitable in such a massive and long-standing institution as the health service. But there has to be time to look at some things and ask whether they are done for the benefit of patients, administrative convenience, or – after all this time – no one at all.

Maybe it seems as if I am asking for jam on it when I know I live in a developed country where good care is mostly free. But I know I am not the only person who believes happier patients live longer and recuperate faster.

From: Caroline, UK

Everything you say is right. I had the same experience nine years ago when my late husband Richard was diagnosed with a brain tumour. We were given the information piecemeal by all the consultants involved and the only person who told me the truth was my GP – I also found out a lot by reading Richard's notes while waiting for a scan. He had

fantastic care from his surgeon
oncologist and neurologist but do you
know the secret? To know as much as they
do! I became a lay expert in brain
tumours and their treatment by spending
hours on the Internet researching medical
and drug sites. Once we could talk in
their language we were treated as human
beings and not statistics.

From: Sue, South Wales

Well done for saying this, Ivan! I have
been an allied health professional for
more than thirty years and a patient on a
few occasions. You've stated exactly what
I have felt and witnessed in my line of
work. Do send this to medical schools. It
is here that our future doctors are
trained. Many new house officers are
arrogant and unprepared for the bad side
of life and ill health. If their bosses
(the consultants) have a poor bedside
manner, as many surgeons especially seem
to have, they need to be taught good
manners and communication skills at med
school.

From: Ellen, UK

As a future doctor (well, come February),
I have taken on board your point.
Throughout my medical training, I have
seen examples of poor communication
skills from highly qualified and

respected consultants. Too bad they give those of us who train in the medical schools of today a bad reputation! We practise communication skills in the safe environment of a videotaped session with actors, and it has been most informative and hopefully will stand me in good stead for the first time I have to tell someone the bad news. However, not all patients want to be fully informed of their situation and some of the skill is in judging how much information is enough for each individual patient.

From: Susan, Scotland

I can remember only too well, that fateful day when I was diagnosed with Hodgkin's lymphoma. The consultant informed me about the disease and that was it. He told me that I would need chemotherapy and radiotherapy and that they would start immediately, but I wasn't informed about anything else. I was completely stunned and I burst into tears when I left the hospital. It would have been so much easier if the doctor had just let me know that they could treat the disease, as I didn't know that then. That was nearly three years ago now, but I still remember it like it happened yesterday.

From: Patricia Evemy, UK

I cannot begin to imagine how the doctors must feel when they have to tell you the news. When I was diagnosed with ovarian cancer, after 'routine' surgery, the doctor told me all the symptoms and sizes of tumour, but couldn't get his tongue around the word 'cancer'.

However, I do know what it felt like to tell my parents, as this task was left to me and in a lot of ways, looking back on it, I was grateful for that. That is not to take away from the fact that seventeen years later, I am still grateful for the prompt action they took to save my life and I too have been blessed with two children they said I would never have after surgery and aggressive chemotherapy. I wish you and your family all the very best; it will be so much easier to tell and hear the good news of the birth of your new child.

From: Jonathan Traynor, Northern Ireland

Spot on, Ivan! After four years working in communications in the health services I can confirm most doctors have the communications skills of a gnat! They are fantastic at their jobs – except when they have to talk to mere mortals about things like prognosis, diagnosis, etc. Even those terms are a mystery to many.

So c'mon, doctor chaps, get some training in basic communications skills.

From: Jenny, UK

I am so glad to read your update. My mother died of a brain tumour some six years ago and the pain we went through was magnified and compounded by her initial consultant's total inability to deliver bad news. What made it worse was that local GPs I spoke to after my mother's death all knew about this consultant's ineptitude but did nothing to address it. Eventually, we found a wonderful neurologist who was able to deliver the bad news in a way that treated my mother with dignity, honesty and, yes, he looked at her and us in the eyes. Maybe you've found a cause where you can really make a difference.

From: Mo, UK

Let's not forget that doctors are human too, who have been patients themselves. It's hard to deliver bad news in any profession.

Reflection – Stephen Kettlewell

I'm a surgeon working in Scotland, and I sent a message to Ivan in July 2004 after he wrote about the difficulties in breaking bad news.

His comments were a useful reminder that what may be another day at work for a healthcare professional is perhaps the most stressful day in the life of the patient. I agreed with him then – and do now – that breaking bad news can be a very hard thing to do.

In my experience, however, most patients seem to know that you are about to give them bad news as soon as you walk into the room. Many of my colleagues would agree with this, and I suspect that it must be down to body language or the patient's own perception of their problem. I have to say that I could probably count on my fingers the number of times people have been completely surprised by what I have had to tell them, although when they have, they have usually been young people.

I have learnt that patients often don't take in much of what they have been told. So I try to be as forthright as possible. It's actually very difficult to look somebody in the eye and tell them that, yes, the results of the tests have come back and that they have shown we are dealing with a tumour. On a human level, telling someone that their hopes and dreams will not come true and that they have an illness which no one in the world can cure is a profoundly tough thing to do.

It's well recognised that there is an 'acceptance curve' with bad news – any kind of bad news, actually, whether it's health or marriage or financial or something else. People will go through denial, anger, depression and may finally end up at acceptance. So we as doctors need to allow people to go through that curve.

One thing I have tried in the past is to record the 'bad news' consultation on tape and give it to the patient who can then go over the details later, since most information given subsequent to the 'I'm sorry it's cancer' statement is forgotten. Their minds are suddenly racing with thoughts like 'I'm going to die', or 'I'll never go to that family wedding', or worries about how much pain they might have. So at least if they have a tape with them, they can take it home and, when they have had a few hours to absorb the initial information, they can hear the rest of the details again.

People assume the worst – they perceive cancer to be a life-threatening, often fatal, illness, and unfortunately that's largely true. This sometimes means that doctors sweep it under the carpet and aren't as clear with patients as they could be. It's not true across the board, and I think the norm nowadays would be to be as clear with patients as possible, but a lot of doctors do obscure what they are trying to say.

Having said that, I have seen patients with abysmal tumours who have made remarkable recoveries. I suspect this is one of the reasons some doctors are tempted to err on the side of optimism when giving bad news – simply because the person sitting in front of them could be the one patient in ten with that kind of cancer who will live beyond five years.

Cancer is cruel because it tells us something about the future. Anyone could wake up in the middle of the night and have a heart attack. But cancer gives you a vision of what is to come that you would not otherwise know about.

It can, however, be used to empower patients.

A colleague had a patient, a young woman who had a cancer from which she was going to die. Ivan has written about how life expectancies are calculated, and that nobody really knows how long a patient will live. My colleague explained frankly to his patient how long she might live if her cancer went untreated, and how long she might live if she received chemotherapy. But he also explained the impact that treatment would have on what time she had left.

The woman disappeared, but one morning her mother arrived at the hospital bearing a letter for my colleague, which said the fact he was now receiving it meant she had died. But it also said that in the time since her diagnosis, she had travelled to all sorts of places round the world which she had wanted to visit. She thanked him for being so frank and honest – as it had allowed her to make the most of the time she had.

19
Tiny Hands

Saturday 24 July 2004

Our son was born on Wednesday morning. He seems a healthy and relatively contented little chap. I have just enjoyed an hour of him snoozing on my chest while I try to read e-mails on my mobile phone and jiggle him around a bit whenever he stirs. I am completely in love with him, of course.

Our daughter is keen on 'her' baby, too. We brought her a present from him but she was far more interested in her new brother, kissing him and holding his tiny hands.

Right up to the last minute, I was worried that I would not be well enough to be with my wife during the birth. Two days beforehand, I had a nasty headache which laid me out for two days and had me seriously worried about what was happening. But it disappeared in time and I feel fine now.

I have a long-standing promise to my wife to keep her life and those of our children private and apart from this diary. For that reason I will not go into detail about the lovely little man who has just become an independent part of our lives.

Let me instead express my heartfelt thanks to the midwives on duty on Tuesday and Wednesday in the birth centre at the Royal Free Hospital in London. Their care was excellent, enthusiastic and reassuring, and the environment they created was exactly what we had hoped for.

And the fact that my sister-in-law kept a supply of coffee and muffins coming was just the icing on the cake.

Thursday 12 August 2004

Our son is three weeks old now. Getting to know him has been a joy and I love the quizzical look he has when he opens his eyes. But the time has been especially happy because for once I have not been fretting about milestones I want to achieve.

It would be easy to let myself lapse and begin to create some more. I could think about how much I want to see his first smile, his first crawl, his first steps and hear his first words. But where would that end? With his first day at school? His first day at work? His first child?

Wanting to see him safely born has been such a strain and a worry for me. I really thought that the odds were against me being there at his birth and I was of course worried too about what might happen to him. Now he is fit and well and so, apparently, am I for a while. I am simply enjoying life with him and the rest of the family.

Things will not carry on like that forever, of course. The day these words appear, I will be having my blood test, picking up my chemo drugs and seeing my oncologist about starting what I think is now my fifth cycle of my current round of drug treatment.

Things seem to be going well. I have finally managed to wean myself off the steroids I take to control the tumour swelling and stave off headaches. This is great because it takes a burden off my immune system and lets me try to shift some of the weight I have put on as a result of the huge appetite the pills gave me.

But I know that my oncologist is going to want to give me a brain scan before long. Brain scans, and specifically the bit where you get the results, scare me. I hate them and I hate knowing they are coming. I would much rather have them unannounced and get the results straight afterwards. But that is not the way the world works, of course. Of all the scans I have had, only one has ever been good news – the time when I had my remission confirmed. I have not had one since March.

Now what is likely to happen is that another milestone will go into the diary and I will have to wait for the day to come. The scan itself is not unpleasant apart from the injection halfway through. But the results need writing up by a specialist and sending on to my doctor, which usually takes two days and leaves plenty of time for nerves to fray.

I should stop thinking about it now and go see to my son's nappy instead.

From: Kath Poole, England

Congratulations to you all on the safe delivery of your new baby boy. Good luck and God bless. He has an amazing dad and mum.

From: Rachel Adler, UK

Dear Ivan, many congratulations on your new son. My parents were both recently diagnosed with late-stage cancers. Your diary shows that living with cancer is just that: living, and can still be punctuated with moments of pure joy and happiness. Thank you for taking the time to remind us of that.

From: Carolyn Bissell, UK

I hope the coming nights are peaceful and the days full of joyous gurgles.

From: Amit, London

I am a doctor in London and work with cancer patients every week. We only see a glimpse of their lives and I always try to keep their hopes alive for the future. In my experience, patients who can keep an overall healthier outlook do seem to have better outcomes. Your diary has given me more insight into the lives, thoughts and fears of patients, and I hope that your writings will make me a better doctor to support them in their hour of need. Thank you and enjoy your new son.

From: Charlie, Ireland

From personal experience of hospitals and scans, I know exactly how it feels when dates and appointments play on one's mind and attempt to take your focus off more important things. Try not to let your impending test stop you from enjoying life as it is right now. All you can do is continue to be positive and take each day as it comes.

From: Abigail Cooper, UK

I send all my best hopes and wishes for
your future and that of your growing
family. We recently buried my 17-year-old
niece who had fought osteosarcoma for
eighteen months. Living that period of
time felt like an eternity, but looking
back it was such a short time and one
which was full of hopes and shattered
dreams. Everything that could go wrong
did go wrong. She suffered tremendously
through the horrendous treatment, always
with such a gorgeous and infectious smile
and such dignity and positive outlook.
Life is not the same without her so I
can only hope that you enjoy every
second, as I'm sure you do. Best wishes.

From: Cliff, UK

When I leave the office tonight I'm going
to cook my four-year-old son his
favourite meal, build a Lego rocket with
him and make the most of our lives
together. Be well, Ivan, and thank you -
from both of us.

20

A Target of Years

I have been a cancer survivor now for two years.

On 29 August 2002, I found out I had a type of brain tumour called a high-grade glioma. As the uncomfortable young doctor who gave me the news put it, 'There aren't any good brain tumours to have, but even if there were, yours wouldn't be one of them.'

It did more than ruin a good August Bank Holiday which I should have spent at a wedding. It turned my life and that of my family upside down.

Since then we have been through a lot. My girlfriend became my wife and has shared joy and sorrow with me, always finding hope in the blackest of days. My seven-month-old baby girl has become a fascinating, charming, hilarious and strong-willed two-and-a-half-year-old ('nearly three', she would prefer).

And after much soul-searching, my wife and I took the decision over a year ago to try to have another child, now our five-week-old son. My diagnosis was followed by a huge dose of radiotherapy. We managed to get married before I moved on to four months of follow-on chemotherapy.

And after all that we had the blessed relief of knowing that I was in remission. With my kind of problem, remissions do not tend to last forever, and head problems came back all too quickly. I had major brain surgery to remove the growing nastiness and implant a new form of chemotherapy drug.

I just made it out of the hospital in time for our first wedding anniversary.

Three months later I was back under the knife to remove another lump of cancerous gunk from my head. After that I thought I was on the way out, but six months have passed and I am doing very, very well, under the circumstances. I cannot concentrate for long periods (but friends would say I never could). I take someone with me when I go out unless I am going somewhere I am very familiar with. I am partially-sighted, having lost my right field of vision to the tumour. My hair will never be the same again.

I have put on lots of weight and rediscovered teenage acne as side effects of steroid medication. I went through a phase of extreme agitation where I was a nuisance to myself and all and sundry.

And earlier this year I got myself as ready as I could to die.

But six months after that last op I feel better than I have for a long time. Maybe I have entered the second remission my cancer specialist told me he intended to give me. I have learned not to think too much about the future. I have tried to live with fear and not surrender to its quiet, corrosive, spirit-sapping power.

I have learned that even with a disease like mine, incurable but sometimes manageable, there are still times when things are getting better. Today's happinesses create the momentum for tomorrow.

We have accumulated two years of survival from single days and weeks, all of which drew heavily on our strength and will. I am so used to living in the short term now that I cannot begin to conceive in real terms of a life beyond the end of the year.

But the most optimistic of my doctors talks now of a 'target of years'. I will do what I can to carry on piling up the days and weeks. It is not easy, but I have learned how by now.

And I will have a quiet sniffle of relief and joy when I see 'nearly three' become really three.

21

The Recurring 'Why?'

Thursday 23 September 2004

Reading *New Scientist* magazine a couple of weeks ago reminded me of something. Back in the mists of time when we evolved consciousness, we understood in a way no other animal did that we were mortal. We grasped the fact that all this activity will, before long, come to an end.

And with that knowledge, we had to evolve a way of putting it out of our minds. Thinking of impending death all the time is a sure-fire route to depression – not much use when you are fighting for survival in a world populated by scary wild animals and a worrying lack of restaurants.

So what I have had to learn – the art of living for the moment in order to make life bearable, cheerful even – is nothing special. But I still have not cracked it 100 per cent.

I cannot completely abandon thinking ahead. What would it be like to be able to think about moving house, or about taking our daughter and son to school?

The fact is that I feel as well as I have done for a long time right now. I am enjoying life and I want more of it. Six months ago things looked very black, yet I was very lucky. The endgame is still the same but I feel as if it is further away than before. And so I want to do something to help myself.

One of the most frustrating things about this disease is the feeling of powerlessness. I want to take charge of the situation and respond to the enormous challenge cancer poses but I do not know what to do next. I am confident that my doctors have given me excellent treatment, but there has to be something I can do beyond taking the medicine and trying to get some exercise.

It would be false of me now to start praying, despite being very grateful for the many prayers I know people have said for me. But my mind remains open to the possibilities of complementary therapies. The problem is that there is so much on offer and so little in the way of quality control.

Obviously it is easy to go for things that do not cost very much, involve little effort and at worst are simply harmless.

I take some ayurvedic herbs every day and I am about to start taking a homeopathic cancer remedy. I'm talking to a French practitioner at the end of October about ways of stimulating the immune system. And I made a firm decision against apricot kernel therapy on the basis that there were as many voices against it as for it and some worrying concerns about possible harm.

But none of these decisions are really based on good science. I have plumped for things where I had a good feeling. Who knows whether they will help? I have shunned things where their proponents have seemed just too insistent or fanatically convinced.

But where are the studies and the randomised trials? Are they even possible? If I could find anything which would give me even a week more in good health then I would grab it, but I cannot try everything and do not want to.

I have had 101 recommendations over these past two years.

But as yet I have found nothing better than gut feeling to guide me. There has to be more.

Tuesday 19 October 2004

Our daughter has discovered the delights of the recurring 'why?'

'Why are we going on the bus?'

'Because we'll get wet if we don't.'

'Why will we get wet?'

'Because it's raining.'

'Why is it raining?'

Other parents must know the routine. You provide a simple piece of information in answer to a simple question and the next minute you are fighting the urge to launch into an explanation of humidity, rainfall and the weather cycle.

Most of the time it is fun. I love how she soaks up information. But some of these queries are starting to lead to answers I do not know how best to handle.

'Granddad is my daddy's daddy!' she announces gleefully one day.

Then she turns to my father and asks him: 'Where's your daddy?'

'Gone,' says my father.

'Where?' she wants to know.

I've been given a book by an Austrian author, Dr Susanne Krejsa, about talking to children about cancer. I cannot pretend I have got all the way through it, but what I have read has really opened my eyes.

Somehow, because neither of my children has ever really been conscious of a time before I had cancer, I have never sat down and thought how, when and what to tell them. But Krejsa makes it clear that children who are not included in their parent's illness quickly suffer. They pick up on all the feelings and anxieties but without explanation. The young ones in particular can easily blame themselves. So my wife and I are starting to decide what to tell our daughter.

It's not easy. It's not as if there aren't any other problems to deal with right at the moment.

I have been told about books specially written to introduce children to the idea of loss. But it makes me want to weep to think that she should have to think of such things so early in her life.

However, I think I've read enough now to be convinced that we shouldn't let too much more time pass by.

Tuesday 9 November 2004

On Thursday I got the results of my brain scan back. I am stable, back in remission.

I have no problem with brain scans. In fact I quite enjoy them. For some reason I quite like being in confined spaces, and, as I've written, I like the noise the MRI machine makes.

But I am terrified of going for the results.

This time it was not as bad as normal. We had taken our son along and he was keeping us and the rest of the assembled company entertained. When my oncologist gave us the news, it was better than we could have hoped for.

I would have been happy to hear that I was to continue on chemotherapy, which I thought the most likely option. I was afraid that after various bouts of headaches and a lot of fatigue I would be told things had got worse and that I might need another operation.

But instead he told me that things were stable, that I should come off chemo and get another scan in four to six months.

I saw my neurosurgeon an hour later and he agreed. 'Go out and live a normal life,' he said.

Last time I heard those words was in January 2003, I think. That seems like half a lifetime away.

I am exhausted. All the tension I had been bottling up as the date and time approached has drained out of me and I feel like someone who has climbed a mountain, come back down again and then cried for an hour at the bottom.

I have all kinds of things wrong with me. My sight will never get better, my hearing is starting to go on one side, and my ability to read and write is starting to play tricks on me.

When I plucked up the courage to look at the scan myself this time, I saw that where the bit of brain which controlled my right visual field used to be is now a hole full of water. It is a strange sight.

But I hear those words 'stable' and 'remission' and I feel so relieved I want to sleep for a week. I might even risk the first beer in six months.

It is wonderful news. We can start making plans again.

22
Life's Cruel Tricks

Tuesday 25 November 2004

Last year we celebrated our first wedding anniversary only a day after I got out of hospital. This year on Tuesday we planned an altogether calmer affair to celebrate our second. It was not to be.

I had some unpleasant but brief headaches over the weekend. Then Tuesday came and things got really nasty. The headache became constant and the pressure in my head was strong. I could not think straight. I had trouble finding simple words and all I wanted was to lie down and for the pain to stop.

My Macmillan nurse has been here three times now, my GP once, and after talking to my oncologist on the phone we have got things under control. I needed anti-sickness tablets to stop me being sick long enough to keep down a fairly hefty dose of steroids.

The suspicion is that I have had a bleed inside my brain. The fact that it seems to have stabilised and that I can even write these words is a good thing. Now I will see my oncologist on Thursday and see where we go from here.

I should not have spoken so soon about liking the MRI scanner.

It would be terrible, awfully bad luck, if the tumour were on the march again so soon after having such good news earlier this month. I have to hope that it was a bleed, that I am on the mend already and that it does not bleed again. That may well be the case.

I want to get back to enjoying my remission soon. There is Christmas, New Year and a birthday to celebrate soon.

And I already have a ticket to join my brother and his family for Chinese New Year in February. It is a date I do not plan to miss.

Thursday 2 December 2004

I was not 100 per cent happy about signing another twelve-month contract on my mobile phone. It was only two weeks since I had been told I was back in remission.

But I plumped for the new 3G phone the day it came out and wrote a review of it; the first piece of non-cancer writing I have had published for a year.

Maybe I was right to worry about tempting fate. The remission is over, after only four weeks of me knowing about it. My aggressive brain tumour is back in business, expanding into my head and the space left for it by my neurosurgeon's knife last time.

Round three of my slow struggle to stay alive has begun, somewhat sooner than planned. I am back on chemotherapy with the surgeon waiting in the wings in case the tumour does not slow. My oncologist has switched me back to the same chemo I had two years ago – temozolomide.

Dealing with relapse is so much easier now. I was not expecting the blow so soon – and what a cruel one after allowing ourselves to contemplate making a six-month plan – but these days I know the form. Make something out of every day that my strength allows and do not look for certainty ahead because the only certainty for any of us is the end.

I got ready for death once, only to persist. I never trusted myself to believe I would see my son born and yet now I see his gorgeous, gummy little grin every day. Painfully I learned not to mourn the future I might have lost. No one has their future until it becomes their present.

And it has paid off. Our kind has endured hundreds of thousands of years without a guarantee of living for three-score-years-and-ten.

I have been encouraged by my wife discovering a website: www.virtualtrials.com. She has been reading the section on glioblastoma survivors. I have not read it myself – still too chicken – but the message I get from her is that there really are people who travel the road I travel – of illness, recovery and relapse, radiotherapy, chemo and surgery – and keep on going. My cancer is not curable but when doctors try to manage it, it is with no half measures. I am grateful to them and to everyone else so clearly fighting my corner with me.

Monday 20 December 2004

My cancer's third, premature reappearance has been a shocking blow. It has come back with a dangerous vengeance at a time when my family and I had allowed ourselves to begin to relax and consider enjoying an apparent remission. I am proud to look at us a fortnight later and see that despite yet another 180-degree turnaround, we are coping. And better than that, we are coping in spades.

My wife, as seemingly always, quietly shows the strength I cannot comprehend, but marvel at daily. For my part, finally now a calm has set in – shorn of the terror that has plagued me on and off for so long these past two-and-a-bit years. These are tough times, but they are happy times, and whatever the physical progress of the tumour right now, its grip on our spirits is weak. I wish that were all I had to write this week.

It is great when I find this diary difficult to write, because it means nothing has happened and I really have to wrack my brains for something to say.

But life continues to play more cruel tricks. As a fit and otherwise healthy 65-year-old, my brave and beloved father received his own cancer diagnosis a few weeks ago.

I have waited until I had spent time with him, and until knowing the initial outcome of his surgery, before accepting his kind offer of letting me write about him.

When my poor wonderful mother told me what was happening, I almost found myself believing that it really was a cruel joke. Our little girl's granddad, who with Grandma is such a cornerstone in the way we keep our lives going, had felt the hammer blow fall. And now for him too, just as for every one of the cancer survivors, so many people in life, everything has suddenly changed for ever.

Dad's diagnosis was weeks ago, rather than months. The NHS in Leeds allocated to him a very highly recommended surgeon who, of course, was only one person in a great team of professionals and carers who have dealt with him in hospital.

Dad's bowel cancer was dealt with by keyhole surgery – laparoscopy. And ten days ago I wept with joy and relief in my wife's arms as I arrived home to an answering-machine message. Dad's surgeon had kindly not made him wait days for a consultation but had phoned him immediately at home to tell him that the tests on his lymph nodes were clear.

We have a real, believable hope from the surgeon that Dad's cancer was a single localised polyp and has been taken away before it had time to spread.

For lucky people caught early, these cancers can be cured. Cure is of course the magical goal. It is a step further from the management of disease, the long and hard job everyone is helping with as I struggle with the vicious little thing dogging my brain right now. Only the passage of time will answer Dad's question.

He told me that he would swap cancers with me tomorrow. I think most parents would do the same – we are at opposite ends of the cancer nasties and he said he would want it to be me with the good prognosis instead of the really awkward one. But I wouldn't want him to. I have got used to my fight and I am delighted he is doing so well in his.

My parents went back to Leeds after spending a few days in London to celebrate Dad's sixty-sixth birthday with us – really great fun. He is now indistinguishable from his pre-op state, though he has to be restrained from interpreting his 'little and often' eating code as meaning 'as much as I like and whenever'.

Dad and I have had to take on cancer from within. Mum has a husband to worry about now, on top of the son she had to worry about before. And my wife bears the double burden. As a cancer researcher she is conducting a slow, painstaking and vital job. It is one which fascinates her but can be maddeningly puzzling and lead down blind alleys costing months or years. Then she comes home to a husband fighting daily with the reality of what the disease is capable of outside a lab and inside a man's head.

It would be so lovely for us all to set cancer aside for three months and not even be able to comprehend the name. But that is not possible and wishing for miracles is a silly waste of time in precious days. But I believe that cancer is losing.

Cancer succumbs all the time both to the incremental improvements of science and the determination of those of us living and surviving the disease day by day. Cancer will lose and people will win.

Wednesday 29 December 2004

When I wrote the time before last, I gave the awful news I so hoped to keep away in the distance. We had been hoping for a breather – maybe six months of calm before the storm.

Instead there was a cancer relapse so virulent and unexpected that for an instant no one seemed sure what to say. But as I write, 2005 dawns. I have had five weeks to adjust and they feel like months.

We are optimistic about my father's prognosis. He begins chemo on 7 January and we hope fervently that his treatment will go well. But no one is the same again after a cancer diagnosis. Dad's early on the road – I am an old-timer now for what I have.

We all have a lot to deal with. But it is as if life has an automatic sense of scale and proportion. As I write, the number of people known to have died in the tsunami, from Somalia across to Indonesia, appears to be 150,000. Hundreds of thousands more are bound to die in the diseases that follow.

I do not have the life I want. I would love to be able to plan for birthdays and Christmases to come. My daughter is almost three and I still cannot believe she will share her third birthday with me very soon.

But I have hope and joy in the uncertainty. I have great hope and faith that I have much to achieve before the end. How different to those hundreds of thousands struggling to stay alive and those who have to bury the dead.

I reached the age of thirty-five without calamity and only a freak accident of genetics blew me off course. My life now is hard but it is fulfilling and I am happy in my short-term way. The uncertainty of my life is a blessing. I have plans and hopes.

I used to fear I would never see my son's birth. Now there will be a fight but it is one which might still see me show up at his first birthday. How completely different to being in a world where a lack of a warning system meant no one could be warned in time? Everyone should have known the tsunami was coming.

I do not know if science will uncover enough about my cancer to slide the dial just far enough for me. But the technology that could have warned millions about the quake? Well, that already exists.

23
The Time Has Come

Thursday 27 January 2005

This is my last diary. I have written it ahead of time because I knew there would be a point when I was not well enough to continue.

That time has now come.

When I began writing about having a brain tumour, I did not really know why. The personal style of journalism was never something I was particularly attracted to, or even interested in reading.

But when I was diagnosed, I had a strong urge to fight back against what felt like the powerlessness of the situation. I really wanted to try to make something good out of bad.

I was not sure if what I wrote would be any good and I was not sure if anyone would read it but I wanted to try. And I also very much wanted to use the diary to maintain my link with my job if I was not well enough to go to work.

I know now that people have found the diary useful, and it meant a lot to me in particular to know that there were people in a similar situation to me, or caring for such people, who got something out of it.

The regular feedback from dozens and dozens of people every time I have written has been wonderful, especially in real times of crisis. I know that it has kept me going much longer than I would have done without it.

I am grateful to many people and this is probably the time to let them know. My oncologist has been superb in his ability to generate optimism in dark circumstances and to provide me with invaluable respite, as has his colleague my neurosurgeon, who has more than once pulled nasty lumps of cancer out of my head with astonishing skill.

I did not see all the members of the teams involved in the craniotomies I had but I know what a superb job they did and how they kept me in comfort and without pain afterwards. They and all the staff involved in my operations and aftercare were first class.

My GP has been unstinting in his support and without his prompt action at the beginning of my drama I believe I would have done nowhere near as well. The support and professionalism of Macmillan nurses is legendary. Mine has been no exception. I clicked with him the minute I met him.

I would also like to say thank you both to the many colleagues and friends at the BBC who have been such a support and especially to the people who manage the department I work for, for their personal support way beyond the call of duty.

What I wanted to do with this column was try to prove that it was possible to survive and beat cancer and not to be crushed by it. Even though I have to take my leave now, I feel like I managed it. I have not been defeated.

Thank you once again to everyone who helped me and came with me. I know the last phase will not be easy, but I know that I will be looked after as I always have been.

I will end with a plea. I still have no idea why I ended up with a cancer, but plenty of other cancer patients know what made them ill.

If two or three people stop smoking as a result of anything I have ever written then the one of them who would have got cancer will live and all my scribblings will have been worthwhile.

Afterword

Ivan died on 31 January 2005, four days after the final part of his diary was published, and two weeks after his daughter's third birthday. He died peacefully with his wife and parents by his side at the Edenhall Marie Curie Hospice in London, to whose staff Ivan's family are grateful for the compassion and respect they showed.

Many thousands of readers sent in comments, newspapers around the world reported his death, and a motion paying tribute to the inspiration he provided was tabled in the House of Commons. Below is a tiny selection of the comments the BBC received.

From: Qaiser Bakhtiari, Karachi, Pakistan

```
People like Ivan are real-life heroes. I
am sure he made an impact on the life of
everyone who read his diary. May God rest
him in peace.
```

From: Joanna, London

Having read Ivan's last entry only last week, hearing that he has passed away has left me stunned. Like most of us I always hoped he'd beat the cancer.

From: Tom, UK

Some of Ivan's legacies will be that his diary has raised awareness, brought this disease out in the open, and provided motivation to those of us lucky enough to be alive to fight cancer until it is a disease of the past. Science can do this in time, I think Ivan believed that above all. Ivan's spirit lives on in all those many ways. My thoughts are with his family – may they be as strong as he was.

From: Neil Morley, Liphook, Hants

I was so sorry to see this news. He was a real fighter, and carried on to the last in order to reap as much time with his family as possible, whom he obviously deeply loved. His words put things into perspective for me. I've started keeping fit now, and think of my family as the motivation. One of the biggest reasons for this was reading Ivan's diaries and realising that you shouldn't take for granted that everyone will be there for you tomorrow or indeed vice versa. I hope that when his children are older, they will read these messages, and realise what an inspiration their father has been to so many people.

From: Peter Lockhart, Bangor, N. Ireland

I found this man's commentary to be a massive reality check. We moan at the slightest inconvenience on a daily basis. The world needs to read every word that Ivan penned and to realise that not one of us knows what a day will bring. We need to count our blessings. This man taught me to count mine. Thanks for the memories, Ivan – your wife and children should be very proud of you.

From: Caroline, Dublin

I would like to convey my deepest and most sincere sympathies to Ivan's family. After reading the terribly sad news about Ivan, I returned to lectures with a heavy heart. I felt like somebody close to me had died even though I've never even heard this brave man's voice. He's made a difference in my life and I thank him for that.

From: Maritza, Panama

Ivan, thank you for reminding us that we have only one life and we need to enjoy it and fight every day no matter what we are going through.

From: K. Jeevan, Kuwait

'I have not been defeated.' I think the world should take Ivan's statement from the final entry in his diary as the slogan for all types of cancer. His positive statement at the final reality which dawned on him says it all. May God

rest his soul in peace and give courage
and strength to his wife and family to
live life to its fullest, as I think that
is what he would have wanted of them.

From: Sue Bunce, Salisbury

My husband has Hodgkin's lymphoma and I
am disabled. Ivan's column was very
important to me and gave me hope and
courage. I was very saddened to hear of
his death – he had so much more to give.
But in a short time he has helped so
many. What more could anyone want from
life? I will always remember him.

From: Miranda Benefield, Texas

As I read the end of Mr Noble's diary, my
heart was filled with a bevy of emotions.
His courage and dignity remind us all
about what Martin Luther King Jr said
about the true character of a man only
being revealed in the face of adversity.
Ivan's death is a constant reminder for
parents and families to live each day to
its fullest and to embrace the lives that
we are lucky enough to live.

From: Charles, London

Sad, sad news. This diary has been a
testament to the human condition. Some
days I could hardly bring myself to read
it. There but for the grace of God, or
fate, or just good fortune, go I. Ivan's
columns have changed his readers and, in
this way alone, his experience lives on
through them. He has made a difference.

Acknowledgements

Thanks are due for the support and friendship of many colleagues at the BBC News website, especially Jon Amos, Alex Kirby, Gary Duffy and Pete Clifton.

Many professionals have contributed to my wellbeing. I greatly appreciate the ongoing care of my oncologist Dr P. N. Plowman, my neurosurgeon Mr F. Afshar, my Macmillan nurse Tony Day, my therapist Nicola Haskins and my general practitioner Dr Thomas Strommer. Dr Roger Lichy has made patient efforts on the holistic front. Thanks are due too to the countless members of nursing staff who have taken care of me, especially Jill Ayres at the Royal London and Steve at the London Clinic. The Bristol Cancer Help Centre gave valuable pointers and Simon Watson taught me chi gong.

Hodder's Judith Longman and her colleagues were kind enough to want to turn my online diary into a book. My colleague Giles Wilson set about the task of editing it with enthusiasm and insight. The BBC's Robin Lustig and Jeremy Bowen were generous with their time. Richard Friebe was kind enough to stick to my good side when he took my picture, a crucial kindness to someone who has had serious surgical attention to the upper left occipital. Vera Brüggemann and Ralph Kostrzewa have been both dear and irreverent friends and welcoming hosts for many, many years.

I am enormously grateful to the countless people who took the time to respond to my writing, most especially to those who wrote to describe their own experiences with cancer. Without them a living dialogue would have been but a dreary monologue.

It would not be right to leave unmentioned the many friends who helped me through the dark times and shared the joys of the good.

Barry Wilcox overcame his well-founded loathing of hospitals to come and admire my bandages. Piers Melbourne and Kevin Oliver several times brought cheer to my hospital bed. Jenny Norton never tires of my dramas and woes.

Monica Whitlock taught me more than she probably realises, not least about how to write, and helped me believe someone would want to read the diaries.

Patrick and Christiane Michl were there right from the beginning. Michael Steininger and Barbara Nicke were the rock-solid friends they have always been.

Mark and Alison Flashman and Kathryn and John Ginn spotted when food, respite and company were so critically needed and were on hand to deliver.

Rachel Cooper and Mehmet Sen walked the tightrope of being consultant oncologists and my friends at the same time. I am grateful for their sensitivity.

In Berlin, Kerstin Lehmann and Uwe Happel took us in and gave succour during frightening days.

Michel Gregoire scoured his home country for something that might help my condition.

Jules Horne sent the comforting words of an old friend and writer.

Mary Arnold-Forster gave us refuge in Skye, took me to my

first ever Burns supper and introduced us to Malcolm, who let me sail the much lamented *Spark*.

Tom Mulligan came to make my lunch when I was too confused to do it myself.

Kate Tobin found time for me when time was scarce.

Bobbie and Andrew Fraser gave generous and repeated hospitality to someone they initially hardly knew.

Their son Simon has witnessed over a decade of my crises and foolishness. I am most grateful for his remaining the very dearest of friends.

My sister-in-law Gerhild and her husband Günter have been our generous hosts for countless escapes to Germany.

I am deeply grateful for the unstinting love and assistance of my parents Ray and Kathy, and my brother Ian. I hope that the latter will be able to forgive my grammatical shortcomings.

I sincerely hope that I have not forgotten anyone – there have been so many kindnesses.

Yet even if by some miracle I conquer my disease entirely and live out my three score years and ten, I know I will still never find all the words for all the thanks due to my loving and beloved wife, A.

London, Hallowe'en, 2004

Biographical Details

Ivan Noble was born in Leeds in 1967 and was educated at comprehensive schools in Luton and Leeds before studying German at the University of Aston in Birmingham. He lived in East Germany from 1988 until 1990 where he worked as a translator. After graduation he joined the BBC, initially as a translator, then as a sub-editor in Nairobi, an Internet journalism trainer and a science and technology writer. He lived with his wife and two young children in North London.